HIDDEN WOUNDS

TRAUMATIC BRAIN INJURY AND POST TRAUMATIC STRESS DISORDER IN SERVICE MEMBERS

PUBLIC HEALTH IN THE 21ST CENTURY

Additional books in this series can be found on Nova's website
under the Series tab.

Additional E-books in this series can be found on Nova's website
under the E-books tab.

DISABILITY AND THE DISABLED – ISSUES, LAWS AND PROGRAMS

Additional books in this series can be found on Nova's website
under the Series tab.

Additional E-books in this series can be found on Nova's website
under the E-books tab.

HIDDEN WOUNDS

TRAUMATIC BRAIN INJURY AND POST TRAUMATIC STRESS DISORDER IN SERVICE MEMBERS

JOSEPH R. PHILLIPS
EDITOR

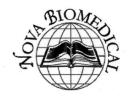

Nova Science Publishers, Inc.
New York

Copyright © 2011 by Nova Science Publishers, Inc.

For permission to use material from this book please contact us:
Telephone 631-231-7269; Fax 631-231-8175
Web Site: http://www.novapublishers.com

NOTICE TO THE READER

The Publisher has taken reasonable care in the preparation of this book, but makes no expressed or implied warranty of any kind and assumes no responsibility for any errors or omissions. No liability is assumed for incidental or consequential damages in connection with or arising out of information contained in this book. The Publisher shall not be liable for any special, consequential, or exemplary damages resulting, in whole or in part, from the readers' use of, or reliance upon, this material. Any parts of this book based on government reports are so indicated and copyright is claimed for those parts to the extent applicable to compilations of such works.

Independent verification should be sought for any data, advice or recommendations contained in this book. In addition, no responsibility is assumed by the publisher for any injury and/or damage to persons or property arising from any methods, products, instructions, ideas or otherwise contained in this publication.

This publication is designed to provide accurate and authoritative information with regard to the subject matter covered herein. It is sold with the clear understanding that the Publisher is not engaged in rendering legal or any other professional services. If legal or any other expert assistance is required, the services of a competent person should be sought. FROM A DECLARATION OF PARTICIPANTS JOINTLY ADOPTED BY A COMMITTEE OF THE AMERICAN BAR ASSOCIATION AND A COMMITTEE OF PUBLISHERS.

Additional color graphics may be available in the e-book version of this book.

Library of Congress Cataloging-in-Publication Data

Hidden wounds : traumatic brain injury and post traumatic stress disorder in service members / editors, Joseph R. Phillips.
  p. ; cm.
Includes bibliographical references and index.
ISBN 978-1-61122-415-3 (hardcover)
1. Brain damage, 2. Post-traumatic stress disorder. 3. Veterans--Medical care. 4. Soldiers--Medical care. 5. Operation Enduring Freedom, 2001- 6. Iraq War, 2003- I. Phillips, Joseph R.
[DNLM: 1. Brain Injuries. 2. Military Personnel. 3. Stress Disorders, Post-Traumatic. 4. War. WL 354]
RC387.5.H53 2010
616.85'212--dc22
                              2010038634

Published by Nova Science Publishers, Inc. † New York

Contents

Preface

Traumatic brain injury (TBI), defined in the medical literature as a disruption in brain function that is caused by a head injury, has become known as one of the "signature wounds" of the wars in Iraq and Afghanistan due to its high occurrence in post-deployment service members and veterans of these wars. As service members return home, many need ongoing care for mild, moderate, or severe TBI. The growing number of TBI patients and the nature of their injuries creates the need for increased treatment capacity for veterans, and raises a number of policy issues that Congress may move to consider. This book provides a review of traumatic brain injury (TBI) as an illness, its prevalence among veterans, current activity to address the issue in the Department of Veterans Affairs, and current policy issues.

Chapter 1- Traumatic brain injury (TBI), defined in the medical literature as a disruption in brain function that is caused by a head injury, has become known as one of the "signature wounds" of the wars in Iraq and Afghanistan due to its high occurrence in post-deployment servicemembers and veterans of these wars. As servicemembers return home, many need ongoing care for mild, moderate, or severe TBI. The growing number of TBI patients and the nature of their injuries creates the need for increased treatment capacity for veterans, and raises a number of policy issues that Congress may move to consider.

In the civilian population, traumatic brain injuries are mainly due to motor vehicle crashes, falls, assaults, and blows to the head. TBI severity may range from "mild," a brief change in mental status or consciousness after the injury, to "severe," an extended period of unconsciousness or amnesia. In addition to physical symptoms, mental health diagnoses such as post-traumatic stress disorder (PTSD), depression, and anxiety are common for TBI patients, as well as substance abuse. Due to the variable nature of TBI injury and recovery, there is not one standard of care or treatment regimen for TBI; patients' needs are diverse, depending on the severity of illness and the presence of co-conditions.

Chapter 2- More than 1.6 million American service members have deployed to Iraq and Afghanistan in Operation Iraqi Freedom (OIF) and Operation Enduring Freedom (OEF). As of December 2008, more than 4,000 troops have been killed and over 30,000 have returned from a combat zone with visible wounds and a range of permanent disabilities. In addition, an estimated 25-40 percent have less visible wounds—psychological and neurological injuries associated with post traumatic stress disorder (PTSD) or traumatic brain injury (TBI), which have been dubbed "signature injuries" of the Iraq War.

Chapter 3- More than 1.6 million American service members have deployed to Iraq and Afghanistan in Operation Iraqi Freedom (OIF) and Operation Enduring Freedom (OEF). As of December 2008, more than 4,000 troops have been killed and over 30,000 have returned from a combat zone with visible wounds and a range of permanent disabilities. In addition, an estimated 25-40 percent have less visible wounds—psychological and neurological injuries associated with post traumatic stress disorder (PTSD) or traumatic brain injury (TBI), which have been dubbed "signature injuries" of the Iraq War.

Chapter 4- REASON FOR ISSUE: This Veterans Health Administration (VHA) Directive defines the policy for the Polytrauma-Traumatic Brain Injury (TBI) System of Care.

In: Hidden Wounds: Traumatic Brain Injury...   ISBN: 978-1-61122-415-3
Editor: Joseph R. Phillips   © 2011 Nova Science Publishers, Inc.

Chapter 1

Traumatic Brain Injury: Care and Treatment of Operation Enduring Freedom and Operation Iraqi Freedom Veterans

Amalia K. Corby-Edwards

Summary

Traumatic brain injury (TBI), defined in the medical literature as a disruption in brain function that is caused by a head injury, has become known as one of the "signature wounds" of the wars in Iraq and Afghanistan due to its high occurrence in post-deployment servicemembers and veterans of these wars. As servicemembers return home, many need ongoing care for mild, moderate, or severe TBI. The growing number of TBI patients and the nature of their injuries creates the need for increased treatment capacity for veterans, and raises a number of policy issues that Congress may move to consider.

In the civilian population, traumatic brain injuries are mainly due to motor vehicle crashes, falls, assaults, and blows to the head. TBI severity may range from "mild," a brief change in mental status or consciousness after the injury, to "severe," an extended period of unconsciousness or amnesia. In addition to physical symptoms, mental health diagnoses such as post-traumatic stress disorder (PTSD), depression, and anxiety are common for TBI patients, as well as substance abuse. Due to the variable nature of TBI injury and recovery, there is not one standard of care or treatment regimen for TBI; patients' needs are diverse, depending on the severity of illness and the presence of co-conditions.

It has been estimated by a recent RAND study that as many as 20% of Operation Enduring Freedom and Operation Iraqi Freedom (OEF/OIF) veterans experience TBI. The Department of Veterans Affairs (VA) has screened almost 250,000 OEF/OIF veterans entering the Veterans Health Administration (VHA) system as of January 2009. As servicemembers return home, these numbers will increase.

VA provides a wide range of services to address the needs of veterans with TBI, including outreach, education, and benefits enrollment information. The FY2010 VA Budget included assurances that VA is working to fund programs that improve veterans' access to mental health services across the country, including those who suffer from TBI as a result of their service in OEF/OIF. In responding to this influx of veterans with TBI and other common OEF/OIF illnesses, policymakers and others have identified areas of concern, including challenges in screening, diagnosis, treatment, and access to care.

This chapter provides a review of TBI as an illness, its prevalence among veterans, current activity to address the issue in the Department of Veterans Affairs, and current policy issues.

Introduction

Traumatic brain injury (TBI) has become known as one of the "signature injuries" of the wars in Iraq and Afghanistan due to its high occurrence in post-deployment servicemembers and veterans of these wars.[1] Soldiers in Operation Iraqi Freedom (OIF) and Operation Enduring Freedom (OEF) are experiencing TBI in large numbers due to blast injuries caused by exposure to improvised explosive devices, rocket-propelled grenades, and mortar/artillery shells.[2] According to one study, among active-duty servicemembers treated at Walter Reed Army Medical Center from 2003 to 2005, nearly 30% of all combat-related injuries included a brain injury.[3] Continuous improvements in battlefield medicine have increased soldiers' survival rates from these attacks. Consequently, increased survival rates necessitate long- and short-term treatment of larger numbers of wounded soldiers.

As servicemembers return home, many may need ongoing care for TBI and related conditions. The growing number of TBI patients and the nature of their injuries create the need for increased treatment capacity for veterans. In responding to these patients, the Department of Veterans' Affairs (VA), Department of Defense (DOD), Congress, and other entities have identified TBI screening, diagnosis, and treatment issues that need to be addressed, including accessibility of care, coordination of care between DOD and VA, and the simultaneous care of TBI co-conditions, notably, post-traumatic stress disorder (PTSD), another common OEF/OIF diagnosis. Congress has allocated significant resources toward TBI research, treatment, and care to address these issues.

This chapter will describe the characteristics of TBI and provide the reader with an overview of current VA activity and key policy issues.

Background

In medical literature, traumatic brain injury is defined as a disruption in brain function that is caused by a head injury.[4] In the civilian population, these injuries are mainly due to motor vehicle crashes, falls, assaults, and blows to the head. Figure 1 shows this distribution. In servicemembers, TBI mainly results from blast injuries caused by exposure to improvised explosive devices, rocket-propelled grenades, land mines, and mortar/artillery shells, as well as motor vehicle crashes, falls, and assaults.[5] The following sections provide an overview of the symptoms and treatment of traumatic brain injury.

Symptoms

At the time of injury, or some time after, TBI could be classified as mild, moderate, or severe.

- Mild TBI may cause a brief period of unconsciousness, mild confusion, or discomfort, while a more severe injury may cause longer periods of unconsciousness, nausea, vomiting, loss of coordination, or other symptoms.[6]

- Moderate TBI may be diagnosed when the patient experiences a loss of consciousness for less than 24 hours, and up to one week of post-traumatic amnesia.
- A TBI injury may be classified as "severe" if it involves more than one day of unconsciousness or more than one week of amnesia.

The perceived severity of the injury depends on a number of factors. Clinically, severity of TBI is measured by the Glasgow Coma Scale,[7] level of unconsciousness, and the extent of post-traumatic amnesia. Physically, the patient may or may not experience structural abnormalities such as skull fracture, bruising, or brain swelling. Trauma may be localized or diffuse, which can result in different symptoms.

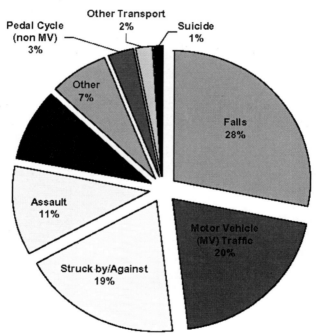

Source: Centers for Disease Control and Prevention, National Center for Injury Prevention and Control, Traumatic Brain Injury, http://www.cdc.gov/ncipc /tbi/Causes.htm.

Figure 1. Causes of TBI in the Civilian Population, 2004

In addition to physical symptoms, mental health diagnoses such as PTSD, depression, and anxiety are common for TBI patients, as is substance abuse.[8] These symptoms may not develop until several months after a head injury.[9] Emotional and behavioral changes are also common and can have lasting effects on interpersonal relationships. Recovery time varies, and some TBI patients have long-term physical effects, including epilepsy and an increased risk for conditions such as Alzheimer's disease, Parkinson's disease, and other neurological disorders that become more prevalent with age.[10]

Treatment

TBI is a complex injury with no specific standard of care or treatment regimen. Studies have shown that patients with mild TBI can make a complete recovery with little or no medical intervention. One study noted that patients with mild TBI recovered more quickly when provided with information on types of symptoms to expect. Other patients need more time and resources, and the nature of those needs varies on a case-by-case basis.[11] In the civilian population, four types of outcomes have been identified for patients with moderate head injuries. Approximately 60% of patients with moderate head injuries make a positive recovery; an estimated 25% will be left with a moderate degree of disability; death or a persistent vegetative state will be the outcome in about 7% to 10% of cases; the remainder of patients will have a severe degree of disability.[12]

Individuals with TBI have diverse treatment needs; treatment ranges in complexity, depending on severity of the injury and the presence of co-conditions. Acute treatment of moderate or severe TBI includes immobilization of the patient to prevent further injury, and immediate treatment of acute physical symptoms. Once TBI patients leave the acute-care setting, some may benefit from a rehabilitation program. The National Institute for Neurological Disorders and Stroke (NINDS) recommends that TBI patients receive an individualized rehabilitation program based upon the patients' strengths and capacities.[13] This program should be adapted over time. Prime candidates for rehabilitation are patients with less severe initial injuries, or those that have started to show significant improvement.

Management of patients with severe TBI requires a coordinated team of specialists, clinical assessments, imaging, and laboratory testing to facilitate recovery. To address both the physical and psychological effects of TBI, treatment and recovery is evaluated by assessments of brain function, functional independence, community participation, and self-reporting of well-being. For more severely injured patients, or for those whose recovery is slow, constant vigilance is required to prevent gradual onset of problems with joint mobility, respiratory status, and many other physiological functions. Patients with mild or moderate injuries, as well as severely injured patients who have improved sufficiently, may be candidates for outpatient therapy. According to the Centers for Disease Control and Prevention (CDC), treatment for individuals who have sustained a mild TBI may include increased rest, refraining from certain physical activities, management of symptoms, and education about what to expect during recovery.

Care and Treatment of Veterans

It has been estimated that as many as 20% of OEF/OIF veterans experience TBI.[14] VA has taken steps to ensure that all veterans are screened for TBI, and that all veterans with TBI are diagnosed and treated. The following sections will describe servicemembers' care and treatment in the VA system, as well as challenges to care delivery for TBI, including the identification of TBI patients through screening and diagnosis, ensuring adequate care for veterans, and ensuring all veterans have access to that care.

As of January 2009, the VA system had screened 249,219 OEF/OIF veterans for TBI. Of those who were screened, approximately 20% (49,297) initially screened positive. Approximately 30,000 of those have completed their comprehensive evaluation, resulting in 13,726 (5.3% of all the veterans screened) confirmed TBI diagnoses.[15] The remaining cases are either waiting to be screened, or have refused further treatment. In comparison to other estimates, this number may seem low. However, this number does not reflect the true prevalence of TBI in the OEF/OIF veteran population for several reasons. Some who screened positive in the initial screen currently are waiting for a comprehensive evaluation, and a small number have chosen not to undergo more testing for TBI. Some servicemembers, particularly those with moderate to severe TBI, are diagnosed by DOD while still on active duty. Additionally, less than half of discharged servicemembers have enrolled in the VA health system and may receive healthcare, as described below.

VA provides a range of services to address the needs of veterans with TBI, including outreach and education, and provides benefits enrollment information to all veterans. For those who are eligible, and who choose to enroll, VA provides screening, diagnosis, treatment, and care coordination services for the veterans, and support services for their families. Veterans generally must enroll in the VA health care system to receive medical care. Eligibility for enrollment is based primarily on previous military service, disability, and income. VA provides free inpatient and outpatient medical care to veterans for service-connected conditions, and to low-income veterans for non-service-connected conditions.[16,17] Additionally, VA has encouraged OEF/OIF veterans to enroll in health services by offering a five-year post-discharge automatic enrollment period for health care. Veterans who enroll during this period are provided care, regardless of service-connected disability status.

Screening

Servicemembers are screened by DOD at discharge and six months following discharge. Following discharge from active duty, a self-administered post-deployment health reassessment (PDHRA) survey is administered by DOD to all servicemembers. This survey includes questions about mental health and TBI symptoms, among other health conditions. However, DOD post-deployment discharge screening of servicemembers may not identify individuals with latent symptoms of TBI.[18] Servicemembers are also screened if they choose to enroll in VA services, and have not previously been diagnosed with a TBI. This section outlines the TBI screening process for veterans.

In April 2007, the VA implemented a policy requiring TBI screening for all OEF/OIF veterans who had not previously been diagnosed with TBI. Prior to that date, TBI screening was not required. The policy coincided with the implementation of a computer-based screening tool with an automated reminder at primary care, dental, and urgent care visits to identify patients at risk for TBI. This reminder, together with reminders for screens for PTSD, depression, alcohol abuse, and infectious diseases endemic to Southwest Asia, constitutes the "Afghan and Iraq Post-Deployment Screen."[19]

Eligible veterans who choose to enroll in the VA Healthcare System are screened for TBI at their initial appointment in the VA system. The screening tool consists of four sequential sections: (1) events, (2) immediate symptoms following events, (3) new or worsening symptoms since events, and (4) current symptoms. The questions in each of these sections are designed to identify exposure to events that increase the risk of TBI. Positive responses at one level open the next section, and negative responses end the screen. If a veteran answers "yes" to one or more questions in each of the four sections, the screen is considered positive, and the veteran is referred for follow-up testing. The follow-up evaluation with a specialist will determine whether the veteran has a TBI or not.

The screening tool currently employed by VA is based on a modified version of the Brief Traumatic Brain Injury Screen (BTBIS), a TBI screening tool used by DOD. Prior to implementation of the modified screening tool, VA did not assess its clinical validity and reliability, which raised questions about its effectiveness.[20] The Government Accountability Office (GAO) raised this issue in a 2008 report on VA screening and evaluation of TBI.[21] In its findings, GAO noted several issues with implementation of the automated reminder and screening tool. Among the issues were a lack of staff training on the tool, and the use of a screening that was modified from DOD's version, but not re-evaluated for clinical validity and reliability. GAO recommended that VA conduct research to assess the screening tool. VA has since undertaken several studies to assess the validity and implementation of the tool.[22]

Diagnosis

For veterans who may have a TBI, but were not diagnosed while on active duty, screening is the first step toward obtaining treatment. However, a positive screen does not conclusively diagnose TBI. The screening tool is designed to be sensitive, to catch all potential cases. Of the nearly 50,000 veterans with a positive screen for TBI, 30,000 had completed their follow-up comprehensive examination as of January 2009, and fewer than 50% of those have been diagnosed with a TBI.[23] Veterans with a positive screen are offered a referral for a comprehensive follow-up evaluation and services with a specialty provider who is qualified to determine a TBI diagnosis.

The delayed onset of symptoms in combination with difficulty navigating the system due to mental health issues may prevent some veterans from seeking treatment. Co-occurrence of psychological symptoms can also complicate diagnosis and treatment. PTSD and TBI have several overlapping symptoms, including insomnia, memory problems, depression, and anxiety, which complicates differential diagnosis and treatment. One study found that 85% of OEF/OIF veterans with TBI had psychiatric comorbidities. PTSD was the most common condition, followed by substance use disorders (26%) and major depressive disorders (19%).[24] In another study, the presence of PTSD in patients with TBI was very strongly indicated by intrusive memories, nightmares, or emotional reactivity.[25] To address the issue of determining the appropriate diagnosis, VA has initiated the Markers for the Identification, Norming, and Differentiation of TBI and PTSD (MIND) study, which will help determine consistent differential diagnostic criteria for TBI and PTSD.

Treatment and Rehabilitation

Servicemembers who sustain injuries receive immediate care on the battlefield, and are then transported to a military medical hospital for treatment. Battlefield treatment may include the removal of foreign bodies, control of bleeding, or craniotomy to relieve pressure from swelling. Once stabilized, DOD can elect to send injured servicemembers with TBI or other complex trauma to VA medical facilities for medical and rehabilitative care. The following sections describe treatment and rehabilitation in the VA system, including a description of ongoing research in these areas.

Many servicemembers who sustain TBI are treated and return to active duty, home, and social responsibilities. Most mild cases of TBI can be resolved without medical attention and may be best served by receiving educational materials.[26] Others may need ongoing treatment and rehabilitation. Outside of the system, VA must work with DOD and other care delivery systems to ensure communication of all relevant information during the transition of care from one entity to the other.

Regardless of the setting, most rehabilitation centers emphasize compensatory strategies, which essentially help patients learn to reach the maximum level of function allowed by their impairments. The concept of cognitive retraining, which presumes that at least some of the brain's cognitive capacity can be restored by constant repetition of certain simple tasks, is emphasized in rehabilitation. Another major goal of TBI rehabilitation is working with patients' families to educate them about behavior they can realistically expect and how they can best help their injured family member. Veterans' care is integrated and coordinated through the Polytrauma System of Care.

Polytrauma System of Care

Many servicemembers are eventually referred to one of the Defense and Veterans Brain Injury Centers (DVBIC), or to a VA Polytrauma Center. The VHA defines polytrauma as "injuries to two or more physical regions or organ systems which occur as a result of the same incident and cause physical, cognitive, psychological, or psychosocial impairments and functional disability." As such, the VA polytrauma system of care is designed to address the multiple types of injuries that occur in conjunction with TBI.

In 2004, Congress passed the Veterans Health Programs Improvement Act. This act directed VA to designate cooperative centers for care of TBI and polytrauma associated with combat injuries. In response, VA introduced the TBI/Polytrauma System of Care (PSC) in April 2005.[27] This integrated, nationwide system encompasses over 100 VA facilities dedicated to serving the needs of servicemembers with TBI and polytrauma. The PSC operates geographically as a "hub and spoke" model with four tiered levels of care. The system is designed to be geographically dispersed, thereby making the specialized treatment requirements of veterans with TBI more accessible.

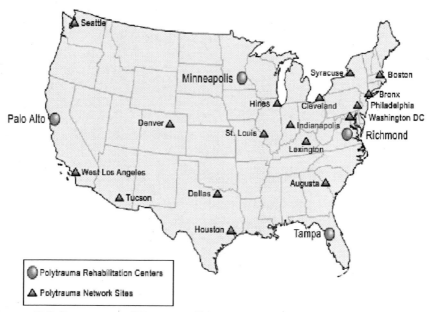

Source: U.S. Department of Veterans Affairs.
Note: A fifth Polytrauma Rehabilitation Center will be located in San Antonio, TX, upon completion.

Figure 2. VA Polytrauma System of Care
Location of Polytrauma Rehabilitation Centers and Polytrauma Network Sites

VA recommends that all veterans experiencing a polytraumatic injury be referred to one of the four[28] Polytrauma Rehabilitation Centers (PRC), the "hubs" of the system. These centers provide acute care for eligible veterans who have sustained severe disabling injuries including, but not limited to, TBI, amputation, visual and hearing impairment, spinal cord injury, musculoskeletal injuries, wounds, and psychological trauma. PRCs provide specific inpatient, transitional, and outpatient rehabilitation tailored to individual patterns of impairments. These centers provide high-intensity care in a residential setting while optimizing the patient's medical condition and improving basic functioning. The interdisciplinary rehabilitation teams include a physiatrist, rehabilitation nurses, occupational and physical therapists, neuropsychologists, recreation therapists, speech-language pathologists, social workers, and vocational counselors.

The PRC provides clinical case management of referrals prior to admission and follow-up case management following discharge. The clinical case manager monitors each patient's progress on medical and functional problems, supports coordination of ongoing rehabilitation care, advocates for the patient's needs, and makes recommendations for alternative care settings when appropriate. Patients are eventually dispersed to the "spoke" facilities, which offer post-acute care, rehabilitation, and care coordination.

Over time, as the patient needs less acute, specialized, or intensive levels of care, VA has tried to make that care more accessible. Polytrauma network sites (PNS), which are located in each of VA's 21 regional health care networks, provide specialized, post-acute rehabilitation for patients who need less intensive treatment, over a longer period of time. They also offer outpatient therapy and day treatment. The next level of care, Polytrauma Clinic Support Teams (PCST), provide facility-based teams with rehabilitation expertise that offer coordination of care, group therapy, and day treatment programs. These therapies address ongoing functional impairments and the management of stable polytrauma conditions.

Every VA facility that is not otherwise designated as a part of the polytrauma system of care has a Polytrauma Point of Contact (PPOC) who is responsible for coordinating the treatment of veterans at their facility. The role of the PPOC is to ensure that veterans are referred to a facility capable of providing the services they require. At all levels of the PSC, the presence of a mental health care professional can be helpful in addressing mental health issues as they arise. VA care of TBI and co-occurring mental health conditions, including PTSD, focuses on reducing functional disability.

Coordination of Treatment

Within the VA, patient care for TBI is tracked through a web-based application that monitors each individual who is screened and referred for comprehensive evaluation and follow-up care. This tracking application is used nationally to capture data on patients who have screened positive for possible TBI, those referred for follow-up evaluation, those who have completed the TBI evaluation, and actions taken to reach those who have not completed the evaluations. The VA creates and distributes monthly reports to assist facilities in developing and refining their clinical processes.

For servicemembers who have been previously diagnosed with a TBI, there may be delays in the transition of medical records from the DOD system to VA due to an identified lack of interoperability of electronic health records between the two agencies.[29] Servicemembers who were diagnosed with TBI while on active duty, in most cases those with moderate or severe TBI, will need coordination of care between DOD and VA. Although progress has been made in this area, it is an ongoing challenge.[30]

The National Defense Authorization Act (NDAA) of 2008 (P.L. 110-181) included provisions known as the Wounded Warrior Act. These provisions were drafted to address congressional concerns about the quality and availability of medical, dental, and mental health services for OEF/OIF servicemembers and veterans.[31] This act required DOD and VA to coordinate research and treatment of TBI and other conditions, and to plan for and evaluate the seamless transition of servicemembers to the veterans health care system. This act also required the VA to establish a rehabilitation and reintegration plan for every servicemember or veteran who receives care for TBI, based on a comprehensive assessment of physical, cognitive, vocational, neuropsychological, and social impairments. Each veteran is assigned a case manager who is required to facilitate implementation of each plan and coordination of care with family members and/or legal guardians involved in developing the plan as much as possible. VA was also authorized through this act to utilize non-VA facilities to deliver the necessary care for servicemembers and veterans with TBI. The act also required the Secretaries of DOD and VA to ensure that TBI victims receive a TBI-specific medical designation, rather than a generic disease classification. This issue was addressed with a revision of diagnostic codes, which are currently being implemented.

Reintegration

Servicemembers with TBI may experience personality and emotional changes after the injury, which may impact their reintegration into family and community life. They experience difficulty with problem-solving, recalling information, and multi-tasking.[32] VA researchers are concentrating on treatment that will improve overall integration and quality of life for veterans with TBI.[33] Researchers have also developed a project exploring community reintegration for servicemembers with TBI to promote seamless transition for those currently being treated, and those who will be treated in the future. Researchers are also assessing which available resources work best to reduce caregiver strains.

Some veterans may qualify for the Federal Recovery Coordinator Program. This program was established in 2008 to address the needs of severely injured veterans who may need additional assistance to obtain the needed level of care.[34] Federal recovery coordinators track the care, management, and transition of recovering servicemembers and veterans through recovery, rehabilitation, and reintegration. This is achieved by coordinating federal health care teams and private community resources to achieve the personal and professional goals of qualifying servicemembers and veterans. Coordinators link servicemembers and veterans with public and private resources, according to their needs. They are assigned to active-duty servicemembers, and continue to assist veterans during and after their transition to civilian life.

Research

The Defense and Veterans Brain Injury Center (DVBIC), a congressionally mandated collaboration of DOD and VA, conducts clinical research on TBI. The DVBIC is composed of a multi-site network, including a growing number of DOD and VA hospitals as well as civilian TBI rehabilitation programs; each site works collaboratively to provide and improve TBI care for active duty military, veterans, and their eligible beneficiaries. DVBIC is currently researching a number of topics, including substance abuse and TBI, a prevalence study of mild TBI, and several studies on neuropsychological function after a TBI.

The 2008 National Defense Authorization Act required VA to establish and maintain a Traumatic Brain Injury Veterans Health Registry, including information on all OEF/OIF servicemembers who exhibit TBI symptoms, and who apply for care or compensation from VA on the basis of any disability. VA is currently partnering with the National Institute of Disability and

Rehabilitation Research (NIDRR) to develop this registry. This registry will facilitate future research by providing longitudinal data on the demographics, military service data, injury information, and treatment of all veterans with TBI. Under the Wounded Warrior Act, VA was also required to implement a pilot program to assess the effectiveness of providing assisted-living services to eligible veterans. The pilot program is ongoing at this time.

TBI is one of the research priority areas for VA scientists. The FY2010 President's Budget request to Congress for VA includes $298 million for TBI research for all veterans, with an additional request for $63 million specifically for OEF/OIF veterans.[35]

Access to Care

Forty-seven percent of veterans from these conflicts have enrolled in the VA system through the third quarter of FY2009.[36] While this enrollment rate of veterans may seem low, it has been increasing since the extension of benefits to five years post-discharge from the military. Additionally, veterans who do not enroll in the VHA system may have health coverage from other sources, such as TRICARE or private insurance. Some who do not receive care may not perceive the need for care due to mild TBI and other, less obvious injuries, including mental illnesses such as PTSD. For others, there may be different barriers to accessing care. Returning servicemembers may not be aware of the symptoms of mild TBI, or the treatments available through the VA. Others may suspect a TBI and/or mental illness, but may avoid diagnosis and treatment due to cultural perceptions of mental illness and potential impact on future employment or enrollment in the Reserves or National Guard. Veterans may be readjusting to life at home after a deployment, and a TBI diagnosis could cause further disruption, including the time and effort required to access treatment, particularly if treatment is not readily available. These potential barriers to accessing TBI diagnosis and treatment are discussed below.

Physical, Financial, and Other Barriers to Accessing Care

To address the issue of low enrollment, and the concern of potential undiagnosed illness due to non-enrollment in VA services, VA has increased outreach efforts to increase awareness of, and participation in, TBI screening of OEF/OIF veterans. The VA provides outreach to veterans during the post-deployment health reassessments (PDHRA) administered by DOD[37] in communities, including DOD post-deployment events, at military treatment facilities and at National Guard and Reserve facilities. Several treatment facilities have contacted veterans to offer screening to those who received care prior to implementation of the VA's screening tool. In these outreach settings, VA staff educate veterans about TBI screening and other benefits.

Veterans may have difficulty keeping follow-up appointments due to work and family commitments, or the lack of nearby treatment facilities.[38] VA has tried to address this challenge through the polytrauma system of care, but some veterans continue to experience barriers to care access. The PSC is designed to be geographically dispersed; however, some have identified ongoing gaps in access to treatment for rural veterans. Some veterans who are recovering from moderate to severe TBI may be best served in a home or residential setting. VA Home Care and Health Services offer in-home rehabilitation on a limited basis for certain veterans who cannot access a treatment center. However, access to local and specialized therapies remains limited. Congress has addressed this issue by providing training and support for family caregivers. Legislation has been introduced in the 111th Congress to further address caregiver support, including training and respite care.

Adequate staffing capacity is necessary to provide an appropriate level of care for veterans with TBI. In the clinical setting, GAO has identified that a shortage of trained staff affects the provision of the recommended standard of care for potential TBI patients.[39] VA clinical providers who administer the TBI screening tool must complete a TBI training module. Some providers who were administering the tool had not completed the required training. One concern raised in the GAO study was a lack of clinical staff to administer the TBI screening tool, and a need for further training on the tool. In response to these findings, VA implemented a TBI screening performance measure beginning in FY2008 to assess the extent of TBI screening for OEF/OIF veterans.

Sociopsychological Barriers

TBI patients exhibit a variety of cognitive and emotional impairments, including attention deficits, interpersonal difficulties, and apathy. Some servicemembers may not be fully aware of behavior changes that result from their injuries. In one study, servicemembers recovering from moderate to severe TBI tended to rate their functioning in these areas higher than close family members rated them, when asked.[40] This lack of awareness of problems can make family support of injured servicemembers even more challenging; the lack of recognition of problems can impede their willingness to get treatment. Additionally, these impairments may compromise servicemembers' capacity to seek care on their own.[41]

Injured servicemembers with cognitive or emotional impairments may have trouble navigating the system that is designed to help them. Veterans with TBI may be eligible for the Federal Recovery Coordinator Program, which helps severely injured veterans navigate the treatment process. Finally, returning servicemembers have work and family commitments to readjust to after being gone several months. It has been speculated that soldiers leaving war zones may minimize or downplay mental health symptoms to avoid any delay in their return home.[42]

Additionally, veterans may not be signing up for VA care because a TBI diagnosis is closely associated with mental illness. According to GAO, there is an ongoing perception that being diagnosed with a TBI would affect veterans' ability to stay in the National Guard or Reserves, or affect other future employment plans.[43] Servicemembers may fear that a TBI is closely associated with a mental health diagnosis, and this could have an adverse effect on future employment, both within and outside of the military.

Finally, there is a perception among OEF/OIF veterans that VA is for the older generations of veterans, and not for veterans of the current conflicts. VA has tried to address this perception through outreach and adaptation of VA services to the needs of recent veterans.

Issues for Congress

As veterans return home from these conflicts, VA has faced an increasing demand for its services, particularly for treatment of "signature injuries," such as TBI. The National Defense Authorization Act (NDAA) of 2008 included provisions known as the Wounded Warrior Act.[44] These provisions addressed congressional concerns about the quality and availability of medical, dental, and mental health services for OEF/OIF servicemembers and veterans. Federal policymakers continue to consider policies and proposed legislative initiatives to address TBI among the veteran population. This section briefly describes policies that Congress may consider regarding support and care of veterans with traumatic brain injury. They are organized into the following topics: (1) identification and screening, (2) continuity of care, (3) staffing and access to care, (4) social and psychological issues, and (5) research.

Identification and Screening

Policymakers have considered whether the current screening and outreach efforts are effective and adequate. Some have raised concerns that VA is not reaching all former servicemembers who may have TBI due to the 2007 implementation of universal TBI screening in the VA system. VA has addressed this concern by initiating a program to contact all OEF/OIF veterans by telephone to inform them of the medical services and other benefits available to them through the VA. The first phase of this program targeted veterans who were sick or injured while in Iraq or Afghanistan, while the second will target all others who were discharged from active duty but who have not contacted VA for services.

Policymakers have also proposed initiatives that would require VA and DOD to coordinate screening and treatment of servicemembers. Some have expressed concern that veterans with mild TBI, in particular, may have difficulty navigating the process of obtaining the appropriate disability status to get treatment, or transitioning from one care system to the other. Programs to ensure the availability of case managers and coordinators have been created for veterans, and some suggest these programs need to be strengthened or expanded.

Continuity of Care

Policymakers and others have expressed concern over the lack of communication of timely and accurate medical information between DOD and VA. The NDAA required DOD and VA to coordinate research and treatment of TBI and other conditions, and to plan for and evaluate the seamless transition of servicemembers to veteran health care systems. This collaboration is ongoing. Policymakers have addressed and continue to assess the ongoing need for VA and DOD to coordinate a continuum of mental health and TBI care for veterans. Congress has proposed legislation to establish a committee that will continually assess VA care for veterans with TBI.

Staffing and Access to Care

The FY2010 President's Budget Request[45] includes assurances that VA is working to fund programs that improve veterans' access to mental health services across the country, including those who suffer from PTSD and TBI as a result of their service in OEF/OIF. Congress has considered legislation that would address the ongoing concerns of TBI treatment and access to care. Many of the measures introduced include funding for PTSD and other combat-related mental health issues, in addition to funding for TBI programs. Some have proposed expanding traumatic injury insurance coverage and benefits to non-OEF/OIF veterans, requiring remote mental health and TBI assessments for veterans without current access to those services through the VA, maintaining benefits for survivors of service members with PTSD or TBI who commit suicide, and providing family caregiver training and support, including respite care.

Congress and VA have considered legislation that would establish pilot programs for servicemembers with TBI to address access issues, including a program to provide training and certification for family caregivers as personal care attendants. Another proposed pilot program would provide respite care by students in graduate programs related to mental health or rehabilitation, and also provide specialized residential care and rehabilitation services for certain OEF/OIF veterans. Other proposals to expand care include further authorization of TBI rehabilitation at non-VA facilities, and the expansion of tele-health alternatives for veterans with TBI and PTSD who live in rural areas. Other proposals would provide training, certification, and support for family caregivers of seriously wounded OEF/OIF veterans, including those with TBI or psychological trauma.

Social and Psychological Issues

Congress has proposed various initiatives for routine TBI and mental health screening for servicemembers, pre- and post-deployment. Congress may review the role of VA and other agencies in servicemember reintegration into work and family life to ensure that social stigma does not provide a barrier to recovery. Other proposed congressional initiatives address potential suicide risks for veterans from OEF/OIF, and address coverage for survivors of suicide victims with combat-related PTSD, TBI, or other mental health issues.

Research

Finally, policymakers have supported increased funding for TBI treatment and research. In FY2009, VA funding for TBI research for all veterans increased by 17% over the previous year; additionally, funding for TBI research for OEF/OIF veterans in FY2009 was increased by 38% over the previous year. Congress has asked VA to conduct research on the following: mild to severe forms of TBI; visually related neurological conditions; means of improving the diagnosis, rehabilitative treatment, and prevention of TBI; and dual diagnosis of PTSD and TBI, and other conditions.

End Notes

[1] Operation Enduring Freedom (OEF) includes operations in Afghanistan and other Global War on Terror (GWOT) operations ranging from the Philippines to Djibouti that began immediately after the terrorist attacks on September 11, 2001, and continue today; Operation Iraqi Freedom (OIF) began in the fall of 2002 with the buildup of troops for the March 2003 invasion of Iraq and continues with counter-insurgency and stability operations.

[2] T. Tanielian, L. Jaycox, ed., *Invisible Wounds of War: Psychological and Cognitive Injuries, Their Consequences, and Services to Assist Recovery*, Rand, 2008.

[3] S. Okie, "Traumatic Brain Injury in the War Zone," *New England Journal of Medicine*, vol. 352, no. 20 (2005), pp. 2043-2046.

[4] T. Tanielian, L. Jaycox , ed., *Invisible Wounds of War: Psychological and Cognitive Injuries, Their Consequences, and Services to Assist Recovery*, Rand, 2008.

[5] Defense and Veterans Brain Injury Center: TBI and the Military, http://www.dvbic.org/TBI—The-Military.aspx (accessed September 14, 2009).

[6] National Institute of Neurological Disorders and Stroke, *NINDS Traumatic Brain Injury Information Page*, http://www.ninds.nih.gov/disorders/tbi/tbi.htm.

[7] The Glasgow Coma Scale is a 15-point scale designed to assess the depth and duration of coma and impaired consciousness.

[8] T. Tanielian, L. Jaycox , ed., *Invisible Wounds of War: Psychological and Cognitive Injuries, Their Consequences, and Services to Assist Recovery*, Rand, 2008, pp. 126-127.

[9] American Association of Neurological Surgeons, "Traumatic Brain Injury," 2007, http://www.aans.org/shared_pdfs/ Guidelines_Management_2007.pdf.

[10] National Institute of Neurological Disorders and Stroke, "Traumatic Brain Injury: Hope Through Research," National Institutes of Health, 2002, NIH Publication No. 02-158.

[11] Veterans Health Administration, *Polytrauma-Traumatic Brain Injury (TBI) System of Care*, Department of Veterans Affairs, VHA Directive 2009-028, June 9, 2009, http://www1.va.gov/VHAPUBLICATIONS/ViewPublication.asp? pub_ID=2032.

[12] American Association of Neurological Surgeons, "Traumatic Brain Injury," June 2006, http://www.neurosurgerytoday.org/what/patient_e/head.asp.

[13] M. Vital, *Traumatic Brain Injury: Hope Through Research* , National Institute of Neurological Disorders and Stroke, Bethesda, MD, September 2002, http://www.ninds.nih.gov/disorders /tbi/tbi_htr.pdf.

[14] T. Tanielian, L. Jaycox , ed., *Invisible Wounds of War: Psychological and Cognitive Injuries, Their Consequences, and Services to Assist Recovery*, Rand, 2008.

[15] Congressional Research Service inquiry to VHA Program Office, January 21, 2009.

[16] The term "service-connected" means, with respect to disability, that such disability was incurred or aggravated in the line of duty in the active military, naval, or air service. VA determines whether veterans have service-connected disabilities, and for those with such disabilities, assigns ratings from 0 to 100% based on the severity of the disability. Percentages are assigned in increments of 10%.

[17] CRS Report R40737, *Veterans Medical Care: FY2010 Appropriations*, by Sidath Viranga Panangala.

[18] T. Tanielian, L. Jaycox , ed., *Invisible Wounds of War: Psychological and Cognitive Injuries, Their Consequences, and Services to Assist Recovery*, Rand, 2008.

[19] Veterans Health Administration, *Implementation of the National Clinical Reminder for Afghan and Iraq Post-Deployment Screening*, Department of Veterans Affairs, VHA Directive 2005-055, Washington, DC, December 1, 2005.

[20] K.F. Carlson et al., "PTSD and Other Psychiatric Comorbidities in OEF/OIF VA Users with TBI," HSR&D Conference Presentation, Baltimore, MD, February 2009.

[21] Congress has mandated in the National Defense Authorization Act for Fiscal Year 2008 that VA and DOD establish a joint interagency program office to act as a single point of accountability in the development of electronic health records systems or capabilities that allow for full interoperability (generally, the ability of systems to exchange data) by September 30, 2009.

[22] Department of Veterans Affairs, *FY2010 Congressional Budget Submission*, p. 87, http://www4.va.gov/budget/ summary/2010/Volume_1-Summary_Volume.pdf.

[23] Congressional inquiry to VHA Program Office, January 21, 2009.

[24] K.F. Carlson, D.B. Nelson, and S.M. Nugent et al., "PTSD and Other Psychiatric Comorbidities in OEF/OIF VA Users with TBI," HSR&D 2009 National Meeting, 2009.

[25] R. Bryant et al., "Post Traumatic Stress Disorder After Severe Traumatic Brain Injury," *Am J Psychiatry*, vol. 157, no. 4 (April 2000).

[26] C.W. Hoge, J. McGurk , and A.L. Thomas et al., "Mild Traumatic Brain Injury in US Soldiers Returning from Iraq," *New England Journal of Medicine*, vol. 358, no. 5 (2008), pp. 453-463.

[27] Veterans Health Administration, *Polytrauma-Traumatic Brain Injury (TBI) System of Care*, Department of Veterans Affairs, VHA Directive 2009-028, Washington, DC, June 9, 2009.

[28] A fifth center is currently in the design phase.

[29] U.S. Congress, House Committee on Veterans' Affairs, *Program Office Improvements Needed to Strengthen Management of VA and DoD Efforts to Achieve Full Interoperability* , Electronic Health Records, 111th Cong., 1st sess., July 14, 2009.

[30] T. Tanielian, L. Jaycox, ed., *Invisible Wounds of War: Psychological and Cognitive Injuries, Their Consequences, and Services to Assist Recovery*, Rand, 2008.

[31] CRS Report RL34371, *"Wounded Warrior" and Veterans Provisions in the FY2008 National Defense Authorization Act*.

[32] S.S. Dikmen, J.E. Machamer, and H.R. Winn et al., "Neuropsychological Outcome at 1-Year Post Head Injury," *Neuropsychology*, vol. 9 (1995), pp. 80-90.

[33] R. Vanderploeg, K. Schwab, and W. Walker et al., "Rehabilitation of Traumatic Brain Injury in Active Duty Military Personnel and Veterans: Defense and Veterans Brain Injury Center Randomized Controlled Trial of Two Rehabilitation Approaches," *Arch Phys Med Rehabil*, vol. 89 (December 2008), pp. 2227-2238.

[34] Department of Veterans Affairs, "VA-DoD Program Serves Severely Disabled Combat Veterans," press release, May 7, 2008, http://www1.va.gov/opa/pressrel/ pressrelease.cfm?id=1499.

[35] VA Department of Veterans Affairs, *FY2010 Budget Submission, Medical Programs and Information Technology Programs*, vol. 2 of 4, May 2009.

[36] VA Office of Public Health and Environmental Hazards, *Analysis of VA Health Care Utilization Among US Global War on Terrorism (GWOT) Veterans*, Department of Veterans Affairs, Washington, DC, October 2009.

[37] Following discharge from active duty, a self-administered post-deployment health reassessment (PDHRA) survey is administered by the Department of Defense (DOD) to all servicemembers. This survey includes questions about mental health and TBI symptoms, among other health conditions.

[35] VA Department of Veterans Affairs, *FY2010 Budget Submission, Medical Programs and Information Technology Programs*, vol. 2 of 4, May 2009.

[36] VA Office of Public Health and Environmental Hazards, *Analysis of VA Health Care Utilization Among US Global War on Terrorism (GWOT) Veterans*, Department of Veterans Affairs, Washington, DC, October 2009.

[37] Following discharge from active duty, a self-administered post-deployment health reassessment (PDHRA) survey is administered by the Department of Defense (DOD) to all servicemembers. This survey includes questions about mental health and TBI symptoms, among other health conditions.

[38] T. Tanielan, L. Jaycox, ed., *Invisible Wounds of War: Psychological and Cognitive Injuries, Their Consequences, and Services to Assist Recovery*, RAND Center for Military Health Policy Research, Santa Monica, CA, 2008, pp 307-326.

[39] U.S. Government Accountability Office, *Mild Traumatic Brain Injury Screening and Evaluation Implemented for OEF/OIF Veterans, but Challenges Remain*, 08-276, February 2008.

[40] R. Vanderploeg, H. Belanger, and J. Duchnick et al., "Awareness Problems Following Moderate to Severe Traumatic Brain Injury: Prevalence, Assessment Methods, and Injury Correlates," *JRRD*, vol. 44, no. 7 (2007), pp. 937-950.

[41] H.L. Lew et al., "Persistent Problems after Traumatic Brain Injury: The Need for Long-Term Follow-up and Coordinated Care," *JRRD*, vol. 43 (2006), pp. vii-x.

[42] T. Tanielan, L. Jaycox, ed, *Invisible Wounds of War: Psychological and Cognitive Injuries, Their Consequences, and Services to Assist Recovery*, RAND Center for Military Health Policy Research, Santa Monica, CA, 2008, p. 7.

[43] U.S. Government Accountability Office, *Mild Traumatic Brain Injury Screening and Evaluation Implemented for OEF/OIF Veterans, but Challenges Remain*, 08-276, February 2008.

[44] CRS Report RL34371, *"Wounded Warrior" and Veterans Provisions in the FY2008 National Defense Authorization Act*, by Sarah A. Lister, Christine Scott, and Sidath Viranga Panangala.

[45] VA Department of Veterans Affairs, *FY2010 Budget Submission, Medical Programs and Information Technology Programs*, vol. 2 of 4, May 2009.

In: Hidden Wounds: Traumatic Brain Injury...   ISBN: 978-1-61122-415-3
Editor: Joseph R. Phillips   © 2011 Nova Science Publishers, Inc.

Chapter 2

Invisible Wounds: Serving Service Members and Veterans with PTSD and TBI

National Council on Disability

Executive Summary

More than 1.6 million American service members have deployed to Iraq and Afghanistan in Operation Iraqi Freedom (OIF) and Operation Enduring Freedom (OEF). As of December 2008, more than 4,000 troops have been killed and over 30,000 have returned from a combat zone with visible wounds and a range of permanent disabilities. In addition, an estimated 25-40 percent have less visible wounds—psychological and neurological injuries associated with post traumatic stress disorder (PTSD) or traumatic brain injury (TBI), which have been dubbed "signature injuries" of the Iraq War.

Although the Department of Defense (DoD) and the Veterans Administration (VA) have dedicated unprecedented attention and resources to address PTSD and TBI in recent years, and evidence suggests that these policies and strategies have had a positive impact, work still needs to be done. In 2007, the Department of Defense Task Force on Mental Health concluded that

Despite the progressive recognition of the burden of mental illnesses and substance abuse and the development of many new and promising programs for their prevention and treatment, current efforts are inadequate to ensure the psychological health of our fighting forces. Repeated deployments of mental health providers to support operations have revealed and exacerbated pre-existing staffing inadequacies for providing services to military members and their families. New strategies to effectively provide services to members of the Reserve Components are required. Insufficient attention has been paid to the vital task of prevention.

PTSD and TBI can be quite debilitating, but the effects can be mitigated by early intervention and prompt effective treatment. Although medical and scientific research on how to prevent, screen for, and treat these injuries is incomplete, evidence-based practices have been identified. A number of panels and commissions have identified gaps between evidence-based practices and the current care provided by DoD and VA and have recommended strategies to address these gaps. The window of opportunity to assist the service members and veterans who have sacrificed for the country is quickly closing. It is incumbent upon the country to promptly implement the recommendations of previous panels and commissions and fill the remaining gaps in the mental health service systems.

In terms of prevention, emphasis must be placed on minimizing combat stress reactions, and preventing normal stress reactions from developing into PTSD when they do occur. When PTSD or TBI does occur, the goal of treatment must be to help the service member regain the capacity to lead a complete life, to work, to partake in leisure and civic activities, and to form and maintain healthy relationships.

PTSD and TBI are often addressed together because they often occur together and because the symptoms are at times difficult to distinguish.

PTSD is an anxiety disorder arising from "exposure to a traumatic event that involved actual or threatened death or serious injury." It is associated with a host of chemical changes in the body's hormonal system, and autonomic nervous system. Symptoms vary considerably but the essential features of PTSD include:

- *Re-experiencing:* Such as flashbacks, nightmares and intrusive memories;
- *Avoidance/Numbing:* Including a feeling of estrangement from others; and,

- *Hyperarousal/Hypervigilance:* Including feelings of being constantly in danger.

The challenge for both professionals and veterans is to recognize the difference between "a normal response to abnormal circumstances" and PTSD. Some will develop symptoms of PTSD while they are deployed, but for others it will emerge later, after several years in many cases.

According to current estimates, between 10 and 30 percent of service members will develop PTSD within a year of leaving combat. When we consider a range of mental health issues including depression, generalized anxiety disorder, and substance abuse, the number increases to between 16 and 49 percent.

Traumatic brain injury (TBI), also called acquired brain injury or simply head injury, occurs when a sudden trauma causes damage to the brain. TBI can result when the head suddenly and violently hits an object, or when an object pierces the skull and enters brain tissue. Victims may have a wide range of symptoms such as difficulty thinking, memory problems, attention deficits, mood swings, frustrations, headaches, or fatigue. Between 11 and 20 percent of service members may have acquired a traumatic injury in Iraq and Afghanistan.

Evidence-based practices to prevent PTSD include teaching skills to enhance cognitive fitness and psychological resilience that can reduce the detrimental impact of trauma. In terms of screening, evidence suggests that identifying PTSD and TBI early and quickly referring people to treatment can shorten their suffering and lessen the severity of their functional impairment. Several types of rehabilitative and cognitive therapies, counseling, and medications have shown promise in treating both injuries.

Service members and veterans may access care through the Department of Defense, the Veterans Health Administration, or the private sector. Each health care system has a number of strengths and weaknesses in delivering evidence-based care. For example:

Department of Defense: DoD has developed a number of evidence-based programs designed to 1) maintain the psychological readiness of the forces in order to reduce the incidence of stress reactions; 2) embed psychological services in deployed settings to ensure early intervention when stress reactions occur; and 3) deliver evidence based rehabilitative therapies on base and through TRICARE, a managed care system that uses a network of civilian providers. However, the military, not unlike the civilian health care setting, has a shortage of mental health providers who must be spread about military bases and deployed settings.

Service members who rely on the TRICARE network may have limited access to services. Because of the low reimbursement rates, many of TRICARE's providers are not accepting new TRICARE patients and because of the shortage of available mental health providers in some areas, enrollees may wait weeks or months for an available appointment.

Veterans Health Administration: VA has undergone significant changes in the past 10-15 years that has transformed it into an integrated system that generally provides high quality care. In response to the increased demand for services to treat OEF/OIF veterans with PTSD, the system has invested resources in expanding outreach activities enhancing the availability and timeliness of specialized PTSD services. Nevertheless, access to care is still unacceptably variable across the VA system.

Some service members continue to face barriers to seeking care. These barriers include stigma and limited access.

Stigma: Service members are affected by three types of stigma:

- Public stigma: The notion that a veteran would be perceived as weak, treated differently, or blamed for their problem if he or she sought help.
- Self Stigma: The individual may feel weak, ashamed and embarrassed.
- Structural Stigma: Many service members believe their military careers will suffer if they seek psychological services. Although the level of fear may be out of proportion to the risk, the military has institutional policies and practices that restrict opportunities for service members who reveal that they have a psychological health issue by seeking mental health services.

Limited Access: Even when service members or veterans decide to seek care, they need to find the "right" provider at the "right" time. Long waiting lists, lack of information about where to find treatment, long distances to providers, and limited clinic hours create barriers to getting care. When care is not readily available, the "window of opportunity" may be lost.

Culturally diverse populations and women face additional barriers. Despite high rates of PTSD, African American, Latino, Asian, and Native

American veterans are less likely to use mental health services. This is due, in part, to increased stigma, absence of culturally competent mental health providers, and lack of linguistically accessible information for family members with limited English proficiency who are providing support for the veteran. Women have an increased risk of PTSD because of the prevalence of Military Sexual Trauma.

Family and Peer Support: Family support is a key component to the veteran's recovery. However, because of the stress of providing care, the veteran's PTSD puts the family at increased risk of developing mental health issues as well. The current system provides inadequate support for the family in its caregiving role and inadequate access to mental health services that directly address the psychological well being of the spouse, children, or parents.

Support from peers who have shared a similar experience is also important. Peers can provide information, offer support and encouragement, provide assistance with skill building, and provide a social network to lessen isolation. Peer support may come in the form of naturally occurring mutual support groups; consumer-run services; formal peer counseling services. In addition, consumers need to be involved in the development and deployment of services for patients with PTSD and TBI.

Recommendations and Conclusion

The wars in Iraq and Afghanistan are resulting in injuries that are currently disabling for many, and potentially disabling for still more. They are also putting unprecedented strain on families and relationships, which can contribute to the severity of the service member's disability over the course of time. NCD concurs with the recommendations of previous Commissions, Task Forces and national organizations that:

1. A comprehensive continuum of care for mental disorders, including PTSD, and for TBI should be readily accessible by all service members and veterans. This requires adequate staffing and adequate funding of VA and DoD health systems.
2. Mechanisms for screening service members for PTSD and TBI should be continuously improved to include baseline testing for all Service

Members pre-deployment and follow up testing for individuals that are placed in situations where head trauma may occur.

3. The current array of mental health and substance abuse services covered by TRICARE should be expanded and brought in line with other similar health plans

It is particularly critical that prevention and early intervention services be robust. Effective early intervention can limit the degree of long term disability and is to the benefit of the service member or veteran, his or her family and society. Therefore, NCD recommends that:

4. Early intervention services such as marital relationship counseling and short term interventions for early hazardous use of alcohol and other substances should be strengthened and universally accessible in VA and TRICARE.

Consumers play a critical role in improving the rehabilitation process. There are many opportunities for consumers to enhance the services offered to service members and veterans and their families. NCD recommends that:

5. DoD and VA should maximize the use of OIF/OEF veterans in rehabilitative roles for which they are qualified including as outreach workers, peer counselors and as members of the professional staff.

6. Consumers should be integrally involved in the development and dissemination of training materials for professionals working with OIF/OEF veterans and service members.

7. Current and potential users of VA, TRICARE and other DoD mental health and TBI services should be periodically surveyed by a competent independent body to assess their perceptions of: a) the barriers to receiving care, including distance, cost, stigma, and availability of information about services offered; and b) the quality, appropriateness to their presenting problems and user-friendliness of the services offered.

8. VA should mandate that an active mental health consumer council be established at every VA medical center, rather than have this be a local option as is currently the case.

9. Congress should mandate a Secretarial level VA Mental Health Advisory Committee and a Secretarial level TBI Advisory Committee with strong representation from consumers and veterans organizations, with a mandate to evaluate and critique VA's efforts to upgrade mental health and TBI services and report their findings to both the Secretary of Veterans Affairs and Congress.

DoD and VA have initiated a number of improvements, but as noted by earlier Commissions and Task Forces, gaps continue to exist.

It is imperative that these gaps be filled in a timely manner. Early intervention and treatment is critical to the long-term adjustment and recovery of service members and veterans with PTSD and TBI. NCD recommends that:

10. Congress and the agencies responsible for the care of OEF/OIF veterans must redouble the sense of urgency to develop and deploy a complete array of prevention, early intervention and rehabilitation services to meet their needs now.

As this chapter indicates, the medical and scientific knowledge needed to comprehensively address PTSD and TBI is incomplete. However, many evidence-based practices do exist. Unfortunately, service members and veterans face a number of barriers in accessing these practices including stigma; inadequate information; insufficient services to support families; limited access to available services, and a shortage of services in some areas. Many studies and commissions have presented detailed recommendations to address these needs. There is an urgent need to implement these recommendations.

Section 1. Introduction

The war is done for me now. The days of standing in the hot desert sun, setting up ambushes on the sides of mountains and washing the blood from my friend's gear are over. The battles with bombs, bullets, and blood are a thing of the past. I still constantly fight a battle that rages inside my head.

Brian McGough, a 32 year-old Army staff sergeant whose convoy was attacked with IEDs in 2006. From his blog "Inside my Broken Skull."

American service members have sacrificed a great deal in the battles in Afghanistan and Iraq, and many of those who have returned are still battling. Only now they are not fighting the enemy around them. They are, at times, fighting an even more elusive foe within—the psychological effects of war. This foe is often not recognized or acknowledged. Moreover, the system that provides treatment for psychological trauma for veterans is not always well implemented.

More than 1.6 million American service members have deployed to Iraq and Afghanistan in Operation Iraqi Freedom (OIF) and Operation Enduring Freedom (OEF), and over 565,000 have deployed more than once (Veterans for Common Sense, 2008). As of December 2008, more than 4,200 troops have been killed and over 30,800 have returned from a combat zone with visible wounds and a range of permanent disabilities (O'Hanlon and Campbell 2008). In addition, an estimated 25-40 percent have less visible wounds—psychological and neurological injuries associated with Post Traumatic Stress Disorder (PTSD) or Traumatic Brain Injury (TBI) (Tanielian and Jaycox 2008; Hoge, et al. 2008).

It is common to make a distinction between visible injuries such as orthopedic injuries, burns, and shrapnel wounds and less visible injuries such as PTSD. The distinction often is characterized as "physical" versus "mental" injuries. These terms imply that PTSD somehow is not physical. However, this is an artificial distinction. PTSD and other "mental illnesses" are characterized by measurable changes in the brain and in the hormonal and immune systems. In this chapter, we use the terms "visible" and "not visible" to make the distinction.

Although PTSD and TBI have different origins—PTSD is caused by exposure to extreme stress, whereas TBI is caused by blast exposure or other head injury—they are closely related. People with TBI are more prone to PTSD, and many people with PTSD may have co-morbid undiagnosed mild TBI. Substance abuse, often associated with both injuries, complicates the situation for many people. Although this chapter focuses on PTSD and TBI, these injuries account for only a portion of the mental health issues affecting our service members including depression, generalized anxiety disorders, substance abuse, and interpersonal conflicts.

War is inherently a traumatic experience, but PTSD can be mitigated through prevention and training programs prior to deployment, effective stress reduction techniques during operations, and treatment programs after combat exposure. DoD, VA, and civilian researchers have developed many strategies to diminish the onset of PTSD and treat both the direct symptoms of PTSD and its impact on the individual's ability to function.

Despite these strategies, a plethora of evidence points to gaps in the current health care system for service members and veterans. Media reports, Congressional inquiries, commissions, and lawsuits have revealed deficiencies in outreach, access, care coordination, and treatment. The evidence points to wide variations in access to mental health services; an inadequate supply of mental health providers; resistance on the part of some military leaders to adopt new attitudes; and resistance on the part of the service member or veteran to seek service because of the stigma associated with psychological disorders.

In the past several years, DoD and VA have developed a number of new programs, policies, and strategies to address the mental health needs of service members and veterans of OEF/OIF. For example, Congress extended the automatic eligibility for services through the Veterans Health Administration from two years to five; DoD instituted mandatory PTSD screening upon service members' return from combat as well as a reassessment 3-6 months later; VA has developed treatment protocols that incorporate evidence-based practices; the Vet Centers have hired additional staff to provide outreach; and DoD and VA are working toward integrating their systems to be more effective.

Although DoD and VA have dedicated unprecedented attention and resources to address PTSD and TBI in recent years (eg. Defense Centers of Excellence), and some evidence suggests that these policies and strategies have had a positive impact, work still needs to be done. In 2007, the Department of Defense Task Force on Mental Health concluded that "Despite the progressive recognition of the burden of mental illnesses and substance abuse and the development of many new and promising programs for their prevention and treatment, current efforts are inadequate to ensure the psychological health of our fighting forces. Repeated deployments of mental health providers to support operations have revealed and exacerbated pre-existing staffing inadequacies for providing services to military members and their families. New strategies to effectively provide services to members of the Reserve Components are required. Insufficient attention has been paid to the vital task of prevention" (US DoD Task Force on Mental Health 2007).

The situation requires an urgent response. While the intensity of combat and the number of enemy initiated attacks has fallen since mid 2007, service members continue to struggle with the wounds of PTSD that they acquired earlier in the war and that others continue to acquire. Early intervention and timely rehabilitation is critical to maximizing the long-term health outcomes of the men and women who served in Iraq and Afghanistan.

NCD's study examines evidence based approaches for prevention, diagnosis, and treatment of PTSD, reviews preliminary indications of many new strategies being implemented by VA and DoD, and concludes that the extra attention being devoted to this disability is not only warranted, but has the potential to greatly reduce financial and human costs for all concerned.

NCD recognizes that these issues have been studied by other governmental and professional organizations. This chapter attempts to augment the recommendations of these previous studies with a focus on barriers to access to care for citizens with disabilities; the importance of early intervention and comprehensive rehabilitation to minimize the long term effects of disability; and the need for continuing consumer involvement both in the rehabilitation of individuals and the oversight of the implementation of the many policy and service delivery changes needed to effectively address the rehabilitative needs of service members and veterans.

This chapter is structured as follows in the succeeding sections:

- Section 2 provides a brief description of the demographic composition of the fighting forces and their experiences in the combat theater. Many of these characteristics are associated with an increased risk of PTSD.
- Section 3 describes the symptoms, prevalence and risk factors for PTSD and TBI.
- Section 4 reviews the evidence-based approaches for preventing and treating PTSD and TBI.
- Section 5 reviews the systems that are in place and discusses how they differ from the evidence based approaches described in Section 4.
- Section 6 addresses the issue of service members not availing themselves of all services.
- Section 7 describes special issues affecting the families of service members and the availability of services to address these issues.
- Section 8 presents NCD's recommendations.

In preparing this chapter, NCD gathered information from scientific journals, professional conferences, commission reports, VA and DoD protocols and regulations, Congressional testimony, newspaper reports, advocacy websites and papers, blogs, on-line support groups, and interviews. These sources represent a range of perspectives including those of DoD and VA leaders, mental health providers, veterans, advocates, parents, and spouses.

Some of the information and recommendations were drawn from the reports of recent task forces and commissions, including the President's Commission on Care for America's Returning Wounded Warriors (the Dole/Shalala Commission); the Task Force on Returning Global War on Terror Heroes (the Nicholson Task Force); the Veterans Disability Benefits

Commission; the Department of Defense Task Force on Mental Health; the American Psychological Association's Presidential Task Force on Military Deployment Services for Youth, Families and Service Members; and, the US Army Surgeon General's Mental Health Advisory Team's annual assessment of needs and survey of deployed troops. A complete list of sources is provided at the end of the report.

Section 2. Background

> *Iraq has become an incubator for post traumatic stress disorder (PTSD) in the American service members. The combat zone in Iraq has no frontline, no safe zone, and the embattled soldier has little with which to differentiate friend from foe, no warning of when or where the next improvised explosive device will be detonated. It is hardly surprising that we are seeing high rates of depression, PTSD, and other anxiety disorders in service members who have been deployed to Iraq.*
>
> Greenburg and Roy, 2007

1. Characteristics of Deployed Forces

The United States has had between 122,000 and 171,000 troops in Iraq and Afghanistan at any one time since major combat operations ended in May 2003 (O'Hanlon and Campbell 2008). Almost 1.6 million American service members have deployed to OIF and OEF, and almost 565,000 have deployed more than once (Veterans for Common Sense 2008).

- 28 percent are guard and reserve (Waterhouse and O'Bryant 2008);
- The average age of an active duty member deployed to Iraq or Afghanistan is 27, and the average age of deployed National Guard or Reserve troops is 33;
- 60 percent of those deployed are married and over half have children;
- 88 percent are male, and 12 percent are female;
- The troops are from diverse racial backgrounds (22 percent African-American, 11 percent Latino, 4 percent Asian, 3 percent other) (Maxfield 2006);

- Half of the 1.6 million service members who have deployed are still in the military (Veterans for Common Sense, 2008); and
- Three-quarters of the forces deployed to Iraq are Army, 15 percent are Marine Corps, and 10 percent are Navy and Air Force (O'Bryant and Waterhouse 2006).

2. Experiences of Deployed Forces

Everyone's experience of deployment is a little different, so it's unfair to cast all experiences in the same mold. People see stories of Infantry guys watching their squadmates die and murdering Iraqi civilians, and assume that I personally have seen levels of Hell of which I have had no taste. Conversely, people read the blogs of career soldiers and Pogues, and perhaps get an image of this place that is a little sunnier than expected. People want to lump our stories into the either/or. All or none. And that's not really fair.
SPC Freeman stationed in Iraq. From his blog "The Calm Before the Sand."

From March 2003 to November 2008, 4,203 American service members were killed in Iraq. Most of the fatalities have been Army soldiers. Forty percent were caused by Improvised Explosive Devices (IEDs), and 30 percent were the result of other hostile fire. Three percent were from car bombs. During intense fighting between May and July 2007, there were 162 insurgent attacks per day with over 75 in Baghdad and Al-Anbar Province alone (O'Hanlon and Campbell 2008)

Many service members are operating under constant threat of death or injury and seeing the violent death of their comrades and others. Enemies and civilians are often indistinguishable, and service members are asked to play dual roles of warrior and ambassador.

Many have been on multiple deployments with relatively little downtime between deployments. Some operations are 24-hours per day with soldiers sleeping an average of only five and half hours per day (US Army Surgeon General 2008). Based on an annual survey conducted by the Army, Soldiers have recently reported a decline in a range of combat exposures. Despite this reduction, the soldiers surveyed continue to encounter intense combat experiences while deployed to Iraq most soldiers have received incoming artillery, rocket or mortar fire. (US Army Surgeon General 2008).

Section 3. Post Traumatic Stress Disorder (PTSD) and Traumatic Brain Injury (TBI)

1. What is PTSD?

The Diagnostic and Statistical Manual of Mental Disorders (DSM-IV), the publication that defines the criteria used in diagnosing mental disorder, classifies PTSD as an anxiety disorder that arises from "exposure to a traumatic event that involved actual or threatened death or serious injury" (American Psychiatric Association 1994).

> *Standing in line at the check out stand the feeling was almost unbearable, like a low electric current was flowing through my body, not enough to hurt but enough to make me really uncomfortable. The people behind me were standing way too close to me, their kid making way too much noise. I thought of the children I had seen in Iraq and how I never saw one cry, even the wounded ones.*
>
> *It felt like I was suffocating in the store, near panic, but I was going to maintain, I could do this, JUST BUY YOUR **** AND GET TO THE CAR.*
>
> *Just then was when the boy behind me popped the balloon he was playing with.*
>
> *I was on the floor, clawing at the fake marble colored tiles, attempting to crawl under a magazine rack. I may have yelled INCOMING I don't know but when I came back into my body everyone was looking at me.*
>
> A 32-year-old OIF Army Veteran. From his blog "This is Your War II."

A. Symptoms

Symptoms vary considerably from person to person, but the essential features of PTSD include the following (description based on Helpguide 2008):

- *Re-experiencing:* The most disruptive symptoms of PTSD involve flashbacks, nightmares, and intrusive memories of the traumatic event. The veteran may be flooded with horrifying images, sounds, and recollections of what happened. He or she may even feel like it is happening again. These symptoms are sometimes referred to as intrusions, since memories of the past intrude on the present. These symptoms can appear at any time, sometimes seemingly out of the blue. At other times, something triggers a memory of the original traumatic event: a noise, an image, certain words, or a smell.

- *Avoidance/Numbing:* Patients with PTSD may attempt to avoid thoughts or activities that could remind them of the traumatic event. In addition, they may lose their ability to experience pleasure and may seem emotionally "flat" or nonresponsive. They may feel detached or estranged from others. Often, they have a sense of a "foreshortened future" feeling that tomorrow may never exist.

- *Hyperarousal/Hypervigilance:* Individuals with PTSD may feel and react as if they are constantly in danger. This increased arousal may disrupt sleep, contribute to irritability and anger, and impair concentration. Hypervigilance may coexist with an exaggerated startle response.

B. The Science

PTSD has a biological basis. It is associated with a host of chemical changes in the body's hormonal system, immune system, and autonomic nervous system. Medical research suggests that the intense bursts of brain activity during traumatic experiences may lay down new neural pathways in the brain (Johnson 2005).

Individuals respond to traumatic experiences along a continuum. Most people have a sudden increased arousal and vigilance. This is a "normal stress response" to danger and generally dissipates with time. For some, the symptoms intensify, become chronic, and interfere with their ability to function (Davidson et al. 2004).

The challenge for mental health professionals and the veterans themselves is to recognize the difference between what has been termed "a normal response to abnormal circumstances" and PTSD. While it is important to avoid "pathologizing" normal reactions, it is equally important to identify when these normal stress reactions are likely to lead to functional limitations. Early intervention will reduce the chance that the stress reaction will become chronic PTSD. In addition, if treatment is delayed, veterans may develop unhealthy coping strategies and may damage their relationships and social support network, leaving them very isolated (Hirsel 2007).

The timing of the onset of stress symptoms varies. These symptoms tend to be heightened by events that elicit memories of the trauma such as anniversary dates or noteworthy "time anchors;" media exposure to war zone events; sights, sounds, or smells that are suggestive of the warzone; certain melodies or lyrics; experiences involving significant losses (such as death of a loved one, etc.); or conflicts with authority (Scurfield 2006).

Some will feel the effects of the trauma while they are still deployed. This is referred to as a combat stress reaction (CSR). Reports from a survey of deployed army revealed that a substantial number of military personnel were experiencing emotional problems during their service in Iraq. For example, 15 percent of those surveyed screened positive for acute stress symptoms and 18 percent screened positive on a combined measure of acute stress, depression, or anxiety. Others may have symptoms immediately upon return from combat, while others may experience a delay of six months to many years, or when they leave the military troops (US Army Surgeon General 2008).

In response to concerns that claims of delayed onset PTSD are attempts to unfairly receive disability compensation, The Institute of Medicine, at the request of the Veterans Benefit Administration, conducted a comprehensive review of the scientific literature and concluded that "considerable evidence suggests that rates of PTSD increase over time following deployment." (Institute of Medicine and National Research Council 2007)

C. Comorbidity

PTSD usually occurs in conjunction with other psychiatric, behavioral and medical conditions. Several studies have found that more than 80 percent of people who have been diagnosed with PTSD also have a generalized anxiety disorder, social anxiety disorder, major depressive disorder, or one of a range of psychiatric or substance-related conditions. (Institute of Medicine and National Research Council 2007). The conditions may be triggered by PTSD (e.g., many people turn to alcohol and drugs in an attempt to self-medicate the symptoms of PTSD), or preexisting disorders may increase the risk of PTSD.

A growing body of research is finding a link between PTSD and poor physical health. People with PTSD have more adverse health outcomes in a number of domains such as self-reported health, morbidity, health care utilization, and mortality (Institute of Medicine and National Research Council 2007). Although the psycho-biological mechanism that causes these adverse general medical health outcomes is not well understood, the evidence of the relationship is overwhelming. For example, researchers have found that compared to veterans without PTSD, those with PTSD have substantially higher post-war rates for many chronic conditions including circulatory, nervous system, digestive, musculoskeletal, and respiratory, even after controlling for the major risk factors for these conditions. (Barrett et al. 2002). They also have found shorter average life spans (Boscarino 2005).

D. Functional Difficulties

PTSD can affect an individual's ability to maintain relationships, work, and in some cases, interact with their environment and those around them.

Relationships: Research with Vietnam veterans clearly documents the adverse effects of PTSD on intimate relationships. Vietnam veterans with PTSD are twice as likely as veterans without PTSD to have been divorced and three times as likely to experience multiple divorces. Veterans with PTSD perpetrate domestic violence at greater rates than comparable veterans without PTSD. (American Psychological Association 2007).

Although many couples are able to withstand the stress of PTSD, some military spouses, in their blogs, describe a similar dynamic. The veteran gets anxious and angry over little things, making everyday life for the family incredibly stressful. Compounding the everyday stress, the veteran may feel emotionally numb and "put up a wall," becoming uninterested in social and sexual activities. The spouse, hurt and stressed, may "snap" at the veteran and the anger escalates as the cycle continues. In other situations, the veteran with PTSD may have a sharp temper or violent streak that scares or angers the spouse.

Work: A diagnosis of war-related PTSD has been linked consistently to poor employment outcomes (Smith et al. 2005). Many symptoms of PTSD can directly affect job performance, such as difficulty concentrating on job tasks, handling stress, working with others, taking instructions from a supervisor, or maintaining reliable attendance.

Interacting with the environment: For people with PTSD, memories may be triggered by sights, sounds, smells, or feelings that remind them of the traumatic event. This reaction may cause them to become isolated.

E. Comorbidity

According to current estimates, between 10 and 30 percent of service members develop PTSD within a year of combat. When one considers a range of mental health issues including depression, generalized anxiety disorder, and substance abuse, the number increases to between 16 and 49 percent (Hoge et al 2004, Milliken et al 2007, Tanielian and Jaycox 2008, US DoD Task Force on Mental Health 2007, Army Surgeon General 2008).

The precise prevalence of PTSD among service members who have returned from deployment to Iraq and Afghanistan cannot be determined at this time. The estimates of probable PTSD are affected by a number of factors including the sensitivity and specificity of the screening instruments used in the study; the time period after combat when the questionnaire or assessment is administered; and response bias among service members who may be reluctant to acknowledge symptoms due to factors such as stigma or fear of impact on their career.

Although estimates vary, all conclude that a significant number of service members and veterans are at risk for various degrees of stress reaction, including for some diagnosable PTSD.

2. What is TBI?

Traumatic brain injury (TBI), also called acquired brain injury or simply head injury, occurs when a sudden trauma causes damage to the brain. TBI can result when the head suddenly and violently hits an object, or when an object pierces the skull and enters brain tissue.

A. Symptoms

Symptoms of TBI can be mild, moderate, or severe, depending on the extent of the damage to the brain. The term "mild TBI" is synonymous with "concussion." (Hoge et al 2008). A person with a mild TBI may remain conscious or may experience a loss of consciousness for a few seconds or minutes. Other symptoms of mild TBI include headache, confusion, lightheadedness, dizziness, blurred vision or tired eyes, ringing in the ears, bad taste in the mouth, fatigue or lethargy, a change in sleep patterns, behavioral or mood changes, and trouble with memory, concentration, attention, or thinking. A person with a moderate or severe TBI may show these same symptoms, but may also have a headache that gets worse or does not go away, repeated vomiting or nausea, convulsions or seizures, an inability to awaken from sleep, dilation of one or both pupils, slurred speech, weakness or numbness in the extremities, loss of coordination, and increased confusion, restlessness, or agitation (National Institute of Neurological Disorders and Stroke 2008).

Most brain injuries are mild, and many soldiers with mild TBI can recover with rest and time away from the battlefield. However, the military estimates that one-fifth of the troops with these mild injuries will have prolonged—even lifelong—symptoms requiring continuing care (US Army Surgeon General 2008). They may have cognitive issues such as difficulty thinking, memory problems, attention deficits, mood swings, frustrations, headaches, fatigue, or many other symptoms.

B. Prevalence

VA only recently began a widespread TBI screening program and DoD has only recently begun documenting TBIs in each service member's medical record. As a result, neither DoD nor VA can estimate the prevalence of TBIs based on screenings. Based on available survey data, an estimated 11 to 20 percent of service members sustained a mild TBI/concussion while serving in OEF/OIF (US Army Surgeon General 2008, Hoge et al. 2008, Taneilian and Jaycox 2008).

3. Relationship between PTSD and TBI

PTSD and TBI are often addressed together for two reasons. First, the symptoms may be similar, so it is difficult to distinguish between the two injuries. Second, many people with TBI also have PTSD.

Although PTSD is a biological/psychological injury and TBI is a neurological trauma, the symptoms of the two injuries have some parallel features. In both injuries, the symptoms may show up months after someone has returned from war, and in both injuries, the veteran may "self medicate" and present as someone with a substance abuse problem. Overlapping symptoms include sleep disturbances, irritability, physical restlessness, difficulty concentrating, and some memory disturbances. While there are similarities, there are also significant differences. For example, with PTSD individuals may have trouble remembering the traumatic event, but otherwise their memory and ability to learn is intact. With TBI the individual has preserved older memories, but may have difficulty retaining new memories and new learning.

Research indicates that people with TBI are more likely to develop PTSD than those who have not incurred a brain injury (Hoge 2008). Two scientific theories attempt to explain this relationship. First, TBI can damage a person's cognitive function and hinder their ability to manage the consequences of his or her psychological trauma, thus leading to a greater incidence of PTSD (Bryant 2008). Second, a mild TBI injury in the combat environment, particularly when associated with loss of consciousness, reflects exposure to a very intense traumatic event that threatens loss of life and significantly increases the risk of PTSD (Hoge 2008).

4. Risk Factors for PTSD

Several factors have been shown to increase the risk of PTSD. Some of these factors are particularly common to the deployments in Iraq and Afghanistan, which may account for the high rate of injury among service members and veterans.

A. *Characteristics of Deployment*

- *Length of deployment*—Numerous studies document a direct relationship between the amount of exposure to combat stressors and the likelihood of eventually developing PTSD (Scurfield 2006).
- *Multiple deployments*—Confirming that the amount of exposure increases risk, the MHAT-V found that soldiers have an increased risk with each additional deployment; 27 percent of soldiers on their third deployment reported serious combat stress or depression symptoms, compared to 19 percent on their second, and 12 percent on their first deployment (US Army Surgeon General 2008).
- *Violation of expectations*—When deployment length is longer than expected (such as when the length of deployment changes in the middle of the deployment) the rate of PTSD increases (Rona et al. 2007).
- *Sleep deprivation*—Soldiers who report being sleep deprived are at significant risk of reporting mental health issues. It is unclear whether sleep deprivation is a symptom or the cause of mental health issues. In MHAT-V soldiers reported an average of 5.6 hours of sleep, which is significantly less than what is needed to maintain optimal performance (US Army Surgeon General 2008).
- *Inadequate dwell time*—The dwell time, (the time between the end of one deployment and a redeployment) has an important impact on PTSD (Hoge 2008) The optimal minimum dwell time for active duty military is twice the period of the initial deployment (a 1:2

deployment to dwell ratio) and a 1:5 deployment to dwell ratio for National Guard and Reserve troops. (Defense Science Board 2007). Thus, a service member deployed for a year should have at least two years dwell time before being redeployed. Many of the adaptive skills necessary in combat must be "turned off" when service members come home and "turned back on" when they return for their next deployment. Evidence suggests that 12 months is insufficient time to "reset" the mental health of soldiers after a combat tour of over a year (US Army Surgeon General 2008).

- *Types of combat exposure*—Certain "malignant" types of combat exposure also appear to place service members at particular risk. For example, McCarroll et al. (1995) found higher levels of PTSD symptoms in veterans who had handled human remains compared to those who had not.

- *Training*—Service members who feel unprepared for their work in theater and those who perceive the events as unpredictable are more likely to develop PTSD (Iverson 2008). Stress-exposure training, which involves simulations of dealing with dead noncombatants, unconventional combatants, injuries, surprise attacks, and live-fire actions, can help prevent combat stress reactions in theater by preparing service members in advance for situations they may face in combat (Hosek 2006).

- *Bodily Injury*—Soldiers who sustain bodily injury are more likely to develop PTSD than are soldiers who experienced the same event but were not physically injured (Koren et al. 2005).

- *Military Sexual Assault*—Being sexually assaulted while in military services leads to PTSD in some, generally female, veterans. There is evidence that military sexual assault makes PTSD more likely than does sexual assault occurring before or after military service (Yeager et al. 2006).

- *Unit Cohesion*—Many researchers have found that strong unit cohesion and leadership reduces the risk of PTSD. High levels of unit cohesion seem to increase the resilience of service members to cope with military-related stressors (Brailey et al. 2007). However, for some, high levels of unit cohesion may be seen later as an illusion that has been betrayed, increasing anger and risk of PTSD (Brailey et al. 2007).

B. Personal Factors

Service members process what happens in combat in the context of the rest of their lives. As a result, early childhood adversity, previous trauma, and history of mental illnesses increase the risk of PTSD. Low education, ethnic minority status, younger age, and lower rank are also associated with increased risk (Brewin et al. 2000, Riddle et al. 2007, Iverson et al. 2008).

Two post-deployment factors are associated with an increased risk of PTSD: lack of social support and "life stress" (Brewin et al. 2000).

Section 4. Evidence Based Approaches for Prevention, Outreach, Assessment, Diagnosis, and Treatment

The goal of PTSD interventions is to address the prevention, diagnosis, and treatment of PTSD. In terms of prevention, emphasis must be placed both on minimizing combat stress reactions, and, when they do occur, preventing normal stress reaction from developing into chronic PTSD. Preventing all cases of PTSD, however, is impossible. When cases do arise, assessment and diagnosis leading to timely treatment is crucial. The goal of treatment is not merely to reduce service members' symptoms, but to help them regain the capacity to lead complete lives as full members of their community – to work, to partake in leisure and civic activities, and to form and maintain healthy relationships with their family and friends.

In an attempt to maximize the effectiveness of their treatment programs, DoD, VA, and the broader psychological community have undertaken studies to identify the best practices for treating PTSD. The "gold standards" for identifying best practices are randomized controlled trials (RCT), which are designed to ensure that any changes in the outcome measure can be attributed to the intervention rather than to extraneous factors. Unfortunately, many promising interventions have not been subjected to RCT studies. In this section, we describe best practices based on theoretical frameworks and medical research in addition to evidence from RCTs.

1. Prevention

Cognitive fitness and psychological resilience can serve as barriers to developing PTSD. Although no RCT studies exist that indicate how to increase this resilience among service members, VA and DoD developed the following general guidelines based on theoretical frameworks (US Department of Veterans Affairs and Department of Defense 2004):

- Provide realistic training that includes vicarious, simulated, or actual exposure to traumatic stimuli that may be encountered;
- Strengthen perceived ability to cope by providing instruction in coping skills;
- Create supportive interpersonal work environments; and,
- Develop and maintain adaptive beliefs such as confidence in leadership, confidence in the meaningfulness of the work, and knowledge about the transitory nature of most acute stress reactions.

Preliminary evidence suggests that psychological preparation enhances resilience. For example, in a 2007 survey of deployed soldiers, those who received pre-deployment "Battlemind" training described in Section 5 reported fewer mental health problems in Iraq than those who did not receive the training (US Army Surgeon General 2008).

2. Outreach, Assessment, and Diagnosis

A. PTSD

Screening: Early identification of PTSD and other stress reactions is critical. Quickly referring people to treatment can shorten their suffering and lessen the severity of their functional impairment.

The effectiveness of screening remains controversial for two reasons. First, screening troops immediately upon return from combat yields false positives, meaning that screening misidentifies cases that are normal combat stress reactions. Medicalizing and pathologizing these reactions may cause the individual to take on a patient role and symptoms that may normally dissipate over time with rest, relaxation, and social support may persist. (DoD response in US Government Accountability Office May 2006).

Second, people may misrepresent their symptoms based on the situation. For example, service members may not admit to symptoms when they are screened immediately upon return from Iraq because they are eager to get back to their families and know that any indication that they need psychiatric help will delay that process. Service members who plan to remain in the military may hide symptoms so that they can stay with their unit. The benefits of PTSD screening 3-6 months after return from combat clearly outweigh the risks. However, the screening does not identify all cases.

Integrate mental health screening and diagnosis into primary care: Because veterans are likely to seek care for a general medical ailment, the primary care physician (PCP) may be the first health-care professional to engage an individual with PTSD. In a study of 103,788 OEF/OIF veterans seen in VA health care facilities between 2001 and 2005, almost one-quarter received a mental health diagnosis and most initial mental health diagnoses (60 percent) were made in non-mental-health clinics, mostly primary care settings (US Department of Veterans Affairs, Office of Inspector General 2007).

The PCP can play a critical role in referring someone to care, but the client may not follow through with the recommendations. There are two models for integrating mental health into primary care that can address this problem. The first is a model of co-located collaborative care between a mental health provider and primary care physician. In this model, if the primary care physician believes the patient has PTSD, that same day she or he can refer the patient to a mental health clinician located in the same building. The second approach is a case management model, in which a primary care physician can refer patients to a mental health provider, and a case manager will conduct ongoing phone follow-up to encourage continued engagement in the treatment process and to assist in negotiating needed adjustments in the treatment plan (US Department of Veterans Affairs, Office of Inspector General 2007).

B. TBI

The best time to assess the impact of TBI is immediately after the injury. For severe TBIs, the impact is obvious and the individual is removed from combat as soon as possible. For mild TBI, many soldiers just "shake it off" but may encounter problems later. Of the three approaches to diagnosing mild TBI, all have limitations. For example:

- **Cognitive Evaluations**—TBI may cause cognitive impairments. Thus, it is useful to measure changes in cognitive functioning. A baseline cognitive assessment is needed so that in the event of exposure to an IED or other types of blasts, service members' cognitive functioning right after the injury can be compared to their baseline functioning prior to deployment.
- **Neuroimaging**—For most mild TBI patients, magnetic resonance imaging (MRI) and computed tomography (CT) scans are inconclusive or difficult to interpret (Belanger et al. 2007, Hoge 2008). Other imaging techniques such as functional Magnetic Resonance Imaging (fMRI), Positron Emission Tomography (PET), and Single Photon Emission Computed Tomography (SPECT) show some promise in detecting mild TBI, but these findings are preliminary (Belanger et al. 2007). Because of their cost, brain scans are not a viable alternative for large scale screenings, but can be useful in some cases.
- **Self-reported History**—Self-reported history of mild TBI/concussion is not well correlated with post-deployment symptoms. Using self reports for screening is likely to result in mislabeling service members as "brain injured" when there are other reasons for their symptoms that may require different treatment (Hoge 2008).

3. Treatment

A. PTSD

Available PTSD treatment can address the primary symptoms of PTSD by helping clients bring under control the vivid re-experiencing of the trauma and the continual re-appraisal of the event so that they can feel better about themselves and their actions. (Brewin 2007). In addition to addressing the symptoms, treatment addresses functional limitations such as relationship and trust issues, anger management, feelings of alienation, sleep disturbances, and other limitations.

In 2004 VA and DoD jointly released a set of clinical guidelines for treating PTSD. The guidelines included individual psychotherapy, group therapy, and pharmacotherapy recommendations based on a review of efficacy studies (US Department of Veterans Affairs and Department of Defense 2004).

1. Individual Psychotherapy

The aforementioned guidelines recommend that the therapist explain to the client the range of available and effective therapeutic options and then the therapist and client should jointly agree on an approach. The guidelines strongly recommend the following four evidence-based practices:

Exposure therapy: The client repeatedly confronts feared situations, sensations, memories, or thoughts in a planned, often step-by-step manner. With repeated, prolonged exposure to previously feared situations, the fear tends to dissipate. ET usually lasts from 8 to 12 sessions depending on the trauma and treatment protocol.

Exposure therapy may be very intimidating for clients to contemplate and can be time consuming and emotionally wrenching for them to complete. The client may have homework in which they write down a nightmare, script a new ending and read the script repeatedly. During the therapy, the client may begin to have more symptoms before the symptoms begin to subside. Thus, it is important to have a strategy to ensure that the client will continue through the entire therapeutic protocol.

In addition, although exposure therapy is highly successful in reducing the key symptoms associated with PTSD, such as intrusive memories, it does not address other issues such as feelings of detachment from others, excessive anger and feelings of alienation. To treat these, the therapist must draw on other therapeutic approaches.

Cognitive restructuring: The client identifies upsetting thoughts about the traumatic event, particularly thoughts that are distorted and irrational, and learns to replace them with more accurate, balanced views. For example, veterans may feel they are to blame for failing to save a fallen comrade even if they did everything they could. Cognitive restructuring helps them look at what happened in a healthier way.

Stress Inoculation Training: This treatment includes a variety of approaches to manage anxiety and stress and to develop coping skills. The client is taught deep muscle relaxation, breathing control, assertiveness, role playing, thought stopping, positive thinking and self-talk.

EMDR (Eye Movement Desensitization and Reprocessing): EMDR incorporates elements of exposure therapy with eye movements or other forms of rhythmic, left-right stimulation, such as hand taps or sounds. For example, in EMDR the client talks about the traumatic event while visually following the therapist's finger back and forth. Eye movements and other bilateral forms of stimulation are thought to work by "unfreezing" the brain's information processing system and allowing the individual to reprocess the memory.

In 2006, the Institute of Medicine (IOM) concluded that, based on results from RCT, the only proven effective intervention is exposure therapy (Institute of Medicine and National Research 2007). The IOM committee noted that this finding does not mean that exposure therapy is the only therapy that should be used. The committee used very strict criteria for evaluating the studies and recognizes that some interventions may be useful but have not been tested. Additional research on evidence-based interventions clearly is needed.

2. Group Therapy

In group therapy, four to twelve clients are led by a mental health professional and can share their thoughts, find comfort in knowing they are not alone, and gain confidence by helping others resolve their issues. Little research has been done to validate its effectiveness, or to delineate those characteristics of group therapy that lead to improved clinical outcomes. The VA/DoD guidelines recommend that this therapy be done in conjunction with individual therapy (US Department of Veterans Affairs and Department of Defense 2004).

3. Pharmacotherapy

In terms of pharmacotherapy, evidence indicates that certain medications, especially selective serotonin reuptake inhibitors (SSRIs) such as Prozac and Zoloft, are effective at relieving core symptoms of PTSD. The VA/DoD guidelines recommend the use of these and several other medications that have shown some efficacy. They recommend against the use of benzodiazepine and typical antipsychotic drugs such as Chlorpromazine, Haloperidol, and Thioridazine.

B. TBI

According to the Centers for Disease Control and Prevention (CDC), treatment for individuals who have sustained mild TBI may include increased rest, refraining from participation in activities that are likely to result in additional head injury, management of existing symptoms, and education about mild TBI symptoms and what to expect during recovery. For some cases, rehabilitative or cognitive therapies, counseling, or medications might be used. Currently, there are no evidence-based clinical practice guidelines that address treatment of mild TBI (US Government Accountability Office Feb 2008).

4. Other Interventions

A. Family Support

Family support is fundamental to a service member's recovery from PTSD. According to a 2005 DoD survey, 74 percent of DoD active-duty personnel cope with stress by talking to a friend or family member (Bray et al., 2006). While there are no randomized controlled studies documenting the value of this informal support, the evidence that does exist suggests this support is extremely important. Spouses and family members are often the first to recognize when service members require professional assistance and often play a key role in influencing service members to seek help (US DoD Task Force on Mental Health 2007).

Unfortunately, this support is not always available. In fact, the very nature of PTSD works to drive this support away. One of the classic symptoms of PTSD is withdrawal, leading veterans to try to shut out the very family members and friends who could help them alleviate their pain. Veterans may be reluctant to open up because they worry that what they say will upset the family. Sometimes when they do turn to their family members, they find that those relatives are under a lot of stress as well, and may not be able to offer needed support.

Providing support and education to the whole family can go a long way toward effective treatment. Family members must be equipped with the ability to recognize distress, and the knowledge of how and where to refer loved ones for assistance (US DoD Task Force on Mental Health 2007).

Family and relationship problems are a serious concern. For example, in a recent anonymous survey of 532 National Guard members, 292 of whom had recently returned from deployment in Iraq, 36% of the deployed acknowledged relationship problems with spouse, 26% relationship problems with children, and 31% emotional numbness that interferes with their relationships. Rates of problems for those deployed were three times greater than for those not deployed. The Army's Mental Health Advisory Team's 2007 surveys indicated that up to 30% of Soldiers and Marines are considering divorce by the midpoint of their deployment, with rates highest for those in their fourth or fifth deployment (US Army Surgeon General 2008). Furthermore relationship problems are a key factor in the majority of suicidal behaviors among active duty service members (US DoD Task Force on Mental Health 2007).

After returning home, relationship problems are often the first symptoms to come to the fore. It is therefore crucial that access to marital and relationship counseling be free of barriers. Early intervention with relationship problems can reduce the long term social costs for veterans and can serve as a means to bring veterans with more severe problems such as PTSD to the attention of healthcare providers.

DoD and VA might consider developing a formal training course for families similar to the Family to Family Education program hosted by the National Alliance on Mental Illness and should continue to utilize the effectiveness of the Chaplaincy Corps.

B. Peer Support

Empirical evidence and theories of PTSD suggest the importance of social support as a moderator of the effects of trauma. Support from peers who have shared the experience is particularly important. Peers can provide information, offer support and encouragement, provide assistance with skill building, and provide a social network to lessen isolation.

Researchers divide peer support models into three categories: 1) naturally occurring mutual support groups; 2) consumer-run services; and 3) the employment of consumers as providers within clinical and rehabilitative settings (Davidson 1999).

Naturally occurring mutual support groups: Service members who return to garrison after their deployment are naturally surrounded by peers. However, this community of peers may not exist to the same degree for National Guard members and Reservists. They receive a short homecoming briefing and usually have 90 days at home before they report back for weekend training. This separation from other soldiers comes at a time when support and connections with others who are going through the same emotional adjustments is critical. This separation may account for some of the increased prevalence of PTSD among the Guard and Reserve.

Consumer-run services: A variety of peer consumer run models exist in the community and in the VA system such as: support groups, drop-in centers, consumer-run organizations; warm lines (peer run telephone call-in service for support and information), and internet support groups and message boards. Research on consumer-run services has consistently yielded positive results.

For example, participants of self help groups have increased social networks and quality of life, improved coping skills, greater acceptance of mental illness, improved medication adherence, lower levels of worry, and higher satisfaction with health (Solomon 2004).

Consumers as employees: In a peer employee model, individuals with mental illnesses are trained and certified and then hired into positions that are adjunct to traditional mental health services. These positions include peer companion, peer advocate, consumer case manager, peer specialist, and peer counselor. Although these models are relatively new, emerging evidence suggests that adding peer services improves the effectiveness of traditional mental health services (Solomon 2004). In addition, the peer provider can alter the negative attitudes of many mental health consumers toward mental health providers, and of some providers toward consumers. In recent years, the evidence for the efficacy and cost-effectiveness of this practice has grown to the point that the Centers for Medicare and Medicaid Services (CMS) has recently allowed Medicaid reimbursement for services provided by peer specialists, and the military in Canada has recently established the Operational Stress Injury Social Support Program based on a peer support model (Veterans Affairs Canada 2006).

Peers may also be used as outreach workers. Service members or veterans who have been deployed during war need not have PTSD or TBI themselves to understand the barriers to seeking services created by stigma and military culture. These peers can help identify people who need professional interventions and facilitate their entry into treatment.

Peer support services should be part of the array of services available. However, if should not be used as a cost-saving substitute for clinical services. As a means of insuring quality care, peer services should implement a credentialing process similar to that of clinical services. Both Georgia and New Jersey have been successful in developing credentialing programs for peer support workers.

Consumers aiding in the development and deployment of services: In order for DoD and VA to develop and deploy services that are responsive to the needs of the consumers, consumers with PTSD and TBI must be included in the planning processes. There are many possible mechanisms. VA has initiated a program for local Mental Health Consumer Councils through which veteran consumers of care, their families and representatives meet with local professional and administrative leaders and assist in identifying problems or gaps in service and brainstorming ways to overcome barriers to care. This program is currently operating only in selected medical centers, and is a local option.

C. Web-based Education and Support

The Internet has become a vital resource for information and interventions. It allows service members, veterans, and their families to access resources immediately and anonymously.

Afterdeployment.org: In response to a 2006 Congressional mandate to develop a website for service members, veterans and their families, DoD has recently unveiled www.afterdeployment.org. The site has 12 modules, each of which address a post deployment issue including adjusting to war memories, dealing with depression, handling stress, improving relationships, succeeding at work, overcoming anger, sleeping better, controlling alcohol and drugs, helping kids deal with deployment, seeking spiritual fitness, living with physical injuries, and balancing your life.

DE-STRESS: VA is exploring the effectiveness of melding an internet-based intervention with professional therapy. In the DE-STRESS program (DElivery of Self-TRaining and Education for Stressful Situations), veterans use a web site to access information and complete a series of homework assignments that monitor, manage and treat PTSD symptoms. The work done on the Web site is self-paced and self-directed and takes approximately eight weeks to complete. The web activities are complemented by either face-to-face meetings or telephone conversations with professional therapists. (Litz et al. 2007).

Other web resources: Websites hosted by a variety of private, nonprofit, and governmental organizations offer easily accessible educational materials such as fact sheets, academic articles, and links to other sources. Two particularly informative sites are VA's National Center for PTSD (http://www.ncptsd.va.gov) and Mental Health America's "Operation Healthy Reunion" (http://www.nmha.org/reunions/info.cfm).

Online support groups offer veterans a relatively anonymous place to share their questions, concerns, frustrations, and fears and hear reactions from people in similar situations. Several MSN groups have emerged such as Iraq War Wives, Aftermath of War: Coping with PTSD, and Iraq War Veterans.

D. Other Nonmedical Interventions

A variety of other nonmedical interventions have shown some promise, but their efficacy is not fully established. These interventions include acupuncture, exercise, and mindful meditation (Hollifield et al. 2007, Stathopoulou et al. 2006, Chartier 2007).

E. Employment and Housing

Veterans with psychological health issues such as PTSD and TBI are at elevated risk of unemployment and homelessness. In addition, evidence suggests that stable housing and supported employment are effective interventions for mental health rehabilitation (Martinez and Burt 2006, Bond 2004). However, availability of housing and employment supports for veterans with mental health issues is limited.

Employment: Individuals with PTSD and mild TBI may have difficulty holding a job. They may, for example, have difficulty concentrating on job tasks, coping with stress, exhibiting appropriate emotions, or controlling anger. In some cases, the employer can make accommodations such as reducing distractions in the workplace, allowing the employee to play soothing music, and allowing flexible scheduling (Artman and Duckworth 2007). In an effort to increase employment options for veterans, the Department of Labor has initiated the "America's Heroes at Work" campaign to educate employers on the issues surrounding the employment of veterans with PTSD and TBI and strategies to accommodate their needs (DOL 2008).

In other cases, the employee may need additional support. Although no employment-related interventions have been developed and tested specifically for veterans with PTSD and mild TBI, promising strategies have been established for people with mental illnesses. For example, substantial evidence indicates that supported employment integrated with mental health treatment is effective in placing and maintaining people with mental health issues in competitive employment (Cook et al. 2005). NCD reviewed strategies for increasing employment among people with disabilities in *Empowerment for Americans with Disabilities: Breaking Barriers to Careers and Full Employment* (National Council on Disability 2007).

Housing: VA has multiple programs that provide short-term housing and treatment for homeless veterans including: the Compensated Work Therapy/Transitional Residence Program; the Homeless Veterans Reintegration Program; the Domiciliary Care for Homeless Veterans Program;

the Homeless Providers Grant and Per Diem (GPD) Program. The Department of Housing and Urban Development (HUD) also assists homeless veterans through a Supported Housing Program funded jointly by HUD and VA and HUD's Section 8 Voucher Program, which specially designates vouchers for veterans with chronic mental illnesses. VA centers also coordinate with local government and nonprofit agencies to assist homeless veterans (US Department of Veterans Affairs 2008).

In 2007, VA estimated that it had served approximately 300 OEF/OIF veterans in its homeless programs and has identified 1,049 more as being at risk of becoming homeless. The experience of Vietnam veterans indicates that the risk of homelessness increases over time. In a survey conducted in the mid-1980's, more than three-quarters of Vietnam-era combat troops and 50 percent of noncombat troops who eventually became homeless reported that at least ten years passed between the time they left military service and the time they became homeless (Perl 2007).

5. Holistic Approach

The Restoration and Resilience Center at Fort Bliss, Texas integrates many techniques described above into one program. The participants are in treatment 35 hours per week for 6-9 months. The treatment includes daily psychotherapy and daily group therapy combined with holistic approaches such as yoga, massage therapy and other nontraditional approaches.

The program also includes a physical component. Participants are required to walk at least 10,000 steps per day, which includes a 45-minute power walk. They also play water polo three times per week, which facilitates their interaction with other people. Throughout the program, the soldiers are also involved in field trips to public places that they might otherwise avoid because they perceive those places as too big, too crowded and too noisy. The soldiers are taught ways to regulate their stress level, so that they can handle the stress of the crowds and noise in these environments.

The program was established in 2007, so its success has not been firmly established. However, early indications are very promising. Among the first set of participants, one-third have graduated and returned to their units, while only two have dropped out and been medically discharged from the Army ("A Soldier's Mind" 2008).

Section 5. Components of the Health Care System

Exhibit 1. Health Care Coverage for Service Members and Veterans

	Active Duty	National Guard and Reserve
Active Duty-Before Enlistment Guard/Reserve - Before Activation	Civilian insurance (private, public, or uninsured) VA or TRICARE for those who are already veterans	
Active Duty Activated Guard/Reserve*	DoD/TRICARE—For troops statio-ned on base, care provided in MTF.	DoD/TRICARE—Most care provided by network providers
Deployment	DoD—In-theater support, embedded mental health professionals, chaplains, etc.	
Post Deployment Deactivated Guard/Reserve	DoD/TRICARE Also have access to on-base military chaplains, family support groups, etc.	DoD/TRICARE—180 days of premium-free coverage. May buy additional 18-36 months for $3,732/yr ($7,984 for family coverage)[1] VA—eligible for enrollment for five years. Once enrolled, eligible for life
After Separation from Military	VA—presumptive eligibility for five years. Ongoing eligibility under certain conditions. Once enrolled, eligible for life. Private Medicare/Medicaid Uninsured TRICARE (under certain circumstances)	VA—presumptive eligibility for five years. Ongoing eligi-bility under certain conditions. Once enrolled, eligible for life. Private Medicare/Medicaid Uninsured

* Guard and Reserve members are considered "activated" when they are called or ordered to duty for more than 30 consecutive days.

As service members move from pre-enlistment, enlistment, deployment, post deployment, and separation from the military, they face a variety of health care systems including the Department of Defense, the Veterans Health Administration, as well as public and private insurance in the civilian sector.

In order to address the needs of all service members and veterans, policy makers must address gaps in all the systems. This section provides a brief overview of the eligibility criteria for each system and the PTSD and TBI services available.

1. Eligibility

Service members (active duty and Guards/Reserves) move through multiple payers and multiple service systems before, during, and after their deployment. At different times they may be covered by Civilian insurance (Medicare, Medicaid, or private insurance), VA, DoD/TRICARE, or they may, at times be uninsured (Exhibit 1).

A. Active Duty
All active duty service members and active Guard and Reserve are eligible for health care through DoD. This includes direct services provided in Military Treatment Facilities (MTFs) as well as a managed care plan (TRICARE) that uses civilian sector providers.

B. Veterans
OEF/OIF veterans are automatically eligible for enhanced enrollment in VA health care services for 5 years with no copayments. National Guard and Reserve members who have left active duty and have returned to their units also receive this enhanced enrollment eligibility. At the end of the five years, these veterans can continue to use VA services, but depending on their income and disability status, they may be required to make applicable copayments.

C. Civilian Systems
Among OEF/OIF veterans who are eligible for VA health care, 35 percent used that care as of December 2007 (Veterans for Common Sense 2008). No information exists on the 65 percent that did not use VA services. Some likely relied on civilian coverage and others may have experienced no perceived need for care. Some may have tried to access VA care, but encountered barriers to accessing services. Others may be unaware of the services that are available. The actual number of eligible OEF/OIF veterans that will use VA services after the 5 year presumptive eligibility period will be determined by service-connected disability ratings and other factors. However, based on an

analysis of veterans under 65, it is likely that a significant majority will rely on private insurance and some will be uninsured (Exhibit 2).

2. Department of Defense

DoD provides health care to over eight million beneficiaries, including active duty personnel, and retirees and their dependents. DoD medical health system (MHS) has two missions—readiness and benefits. The *readiness mission* ensures that personnel are ready to deploy, provides medical services and support to the armed forces during military operations, and involves deploying medical personnel and equipment to support military forces throughout the world. The *benefits mission* provides medical services and support to members of the armed forces, their family members, and others entitled to DoD health care. (US GAO 2007).

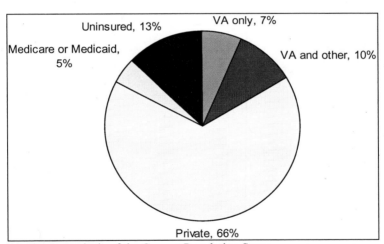

Source: Author's Analysis of the Current Population Survey
Description: Pie chart showing that among veterans under age 65, 17 percent are enrolled with VA (7 percent use VA only, 10 percent use VA in conjunction with other insurance). Most veterans (66 percent) are privately insured and do not use VA, 5 percent are enrolled in Medicare or Medicaid, and 13 percent are uninsured.

Exhibit 2. Health Insurance Status of Veterans Under age 65, 2007

DoD's dual health care mission is carried out through a direct care system that comprises 530 Army, Navy, and Air Force Military Treatment Facilities (MTFs) worldwide. Within the direct care system, each military branch is responsible for managing its MTFs and other activities. Historically, these separate systems are not well coordinated. The services generally fail to cooperate with each other and resist efforts to consolidate their medical departments (US GAO 2007)

DoD also operates a purchased care system that uses civilian managed care support contractors (TRICARE) to develop networks of civilian primary and specialty care providers and to provide other customer service functions, such as claims processing.

Prevention Programs: The Army's signature prevention program is the mandatory Battlemind training program, which is provided in a large group setting to all Army personnel prior to deployment, and immediately upon return. In the 45-minute pre-deployment program, soldiers about to deploy are told what they are likely to see, hear, think, and feel. The post-deployment program explains the possible impact of deployment on psychological, social-emotional, and behavioral functioning. It explains what is "normal" and provides information about available mental health resources available should service members have difficulties readjusting. The Battlemind program highlights the problems that can occur when the skills needed for effective combat are carried over into the home environment (Exhibit 3).

Exhibit 3. Combat Skills that Can Cause Problems if Not Adapted to the Home Front

Combat Skill	Negative Presentation on the Home Front
Buddies (cohesion)	Withdrawal
Accountability	Controlling
Targeted Aggression	Inappropriate Aggression
Tactical Awareness	Hypervigilance
Lethally Armed	"Locked and Loaded" at Home
Emotional Control	Anger/Detachment
Mission Operational Security (OPSEC)	Secretiveness
Individual Responsibility	Guilt
NonDefensive (combat) Driving	Aggressive Driving
Discipline and Ordering	Conflict

Source: Walter Reed Army Institute of Research 2007

Battlemind has shown some success. The Army's most recent survey of deployed soldiers found that soldiers who received training were less likely to screen positive for mental health problems while in Iraq (12 percent compared to 21 percent). Soldiers that did not screen positive were significantly more likely to agree that (a) the training in managing the stress of deployment was adequate, and (b) the training to identify service members at risk for suicide was sufficient. However, even with Battlemind training, one-third of soldiers were not confident in their ability to help service members get mental health assistance, and 40 percent were not confident in their ability to identify service members at risk of suicide (US Army Surgeon General 2008)

Mandatory Behavioral Health Screenings for PTSD: Beginning in 1998, DoD has required service members to complete a Pre-Deployment Health Assessment (PHA) shortly before deployment and the Post-Deployment Health Assessment (PDHA) immediately after deployment. Recognizing that a service member's symptoms may change over time, DoD recently mandated that the Post-Deployment Health Re-Assessment (PDHRA) be completed six months after the service member returns home.

Military members complete a brief set of screening questions, which are reviewed by a mental health professional. The service member is supposed to be referred for additional services as needed. Although the screenings potentially can identify individuals who need, but do not seek, services, they have significant limitations.

- Implementation of this program varies among military installations, and the reviewing providers may lack the necessary training to detect and address pathology (US GAO May, 2006).
- Referrals are inconsistent. A GAO report found that, four of five returning troops potentially at risk for PTSD, were not referred for further mental health evaluation. Half of those eventually got help on their own, but less than 10 percent were referred through the military (US GAO May, 2006).
- Service members may not accurately report their mental health concerns.

TBI Screenings: DoD admits that it lacks a system-wide approach for proper identification, management, and surveillance of individuals who sustain mild to moderate TBI (English 2007). However, quality pilot programs have been in existence for some time and efforts are underway to make screening universal.

Treatment: In addition to services available through TRICARE (described in detail below), DoD has a variety of programs designed to maintain the psychological readiness of the forces that are administered both within and outside the confines of the Defense Health Program including, for example:

- *Military Treatment Facility:* Installation-level military medical treatment facilities and the larger military medical centers and clinics each develop and implement programs focusing on deployment issues. While there are a number of excellent programs, the availability, coherence, and quality of such programs varies across the system, depending upon the number of mental health professionals assigned to the unit, their training and experience, and command support for behavioral health programs (US DoD Task Force on Mental Health 2007).

- *Military OneSource:* This initiative offers a 24-hour, 7-day-a-week, confidential nonmedical information and referral system that can be accessed through the telephone, Internet, and e-mail. It also offers confidential short-term (up to six sessions per year per problem), face-to-face counseling for nonclinical problems. If care is sought for a clinical problem for which TRICARE provides reimbursement, Military OneSource refers the individual to TRICARE or the nearest MTF.

- *Chaplains:* Military mental health services often are delivered in partnership with services provided by military chaplains. This is especially true in deployed environments where mental health and pastoral services constitute an essential component of deployment support. Outside of the deployed environment, military chaplains provide marital and individual counseling, and service members may seek out chaplains because issues of stigma may be lessened, and greater assurances of confidentiality may be offered.

- *Substance Abuse Prevention and Treatment:* Each military service has substance abuse prevention and treatment programs.

- *Other Organizations:* A number of other organizations provide direct or indirect support for the psychological health of military members and their families, including Health Promotions Offices, Sexual Assault Prevention and Response Offices, Exceptional Family Member Programs, Suicide Prevention Programs, and Combat Operational Stress Control programs.

This multiplicity of programs, policies, and funding streams provides many points of access to support for psychological health. However, the multiplicity may also lead to confusion about benefits and services, fragmented delivery of care, and gaps in service provision (US DoD Task Force on Mental Health 2007) and cause considerable variation in mental health service delivery among the different bases and military services.

In addition, the military has a shortage of uniformed behavioral health professionals. This shortage is exacerbated by the need to spread these providers between deployed and nondeployed settings, the high turnover rate, and the limited ability to rely on civilian professionals (American Psychological Association 2007). Several commissions and studies—including the DoD Task Force on Mental Health—have concluded that the number of mental health care professionals in the military health care system is too low to meet current needs.

The military is trying to meet this demand for mental health by offering financial incentives to recruit and retain existing psychologists, psychiatrists and other mental health professionals, and by offering expanding internship opportunities for training. Besides bringing on more professionals to active duty, the Army, Navy and Air Force are all hiring professionals as civilian contractors or federal employees.

Psychological Health Services in Theater: Recognizing that isolating mental health professionals in offices or clinics may discourage service members with concerns about the stigma from seeking care, the military has been embedding mental health providers in units. Each branch has developed a slightly different approach but all are based on the theory that keeping service members with their units helps in the recovery process.

The Army has three tiers of care. The first tier is provided by fellow service members or uniformed mental health professionals and chaplains embedded with the troops. In the next tier, the soldier is taken to a "combat stress control unit" for one to three days of rest, hot food, hot showers, clean uniforms and medication if needed. The stress control unit is near the combat unit and can relocate if the combat unit relocates. Soldiers are treated with the expectation that they will feel better in a couple of days and go back to work. An advantage of this approach is that soldiers maintain their identity with their combat unit and leadership. The third tier is a combat support hospital that provides more intensive services. If the issue cannot be resolved in these settings, the soldier is evacuated to Germany or the United States.

The Marines' Operational Stress Control and Readiness (OSCAR) program matches psychologists, psychiatrists and mental health technicians with Marine regiments in the months before a deployment, continuing during a rotation in Iraq, then back home. The Navy has the "Psychologists at Sea" program that puts Navy psychologists aboard aircraft carriers.

Despite these new programs, access to behavioral health services in theater is limited. Compared to 2006, soldiers reported more difficulty accessing services in 2007. The Army advisory team cites a shortage of behavioral health personnel in Iraq, with one behavioral health provider for every 734 soldiers (US Army Surgeon General 2008).

TRICARE: TRICARE Prime, the health care plan available to active duty service members and activated guard and reserve troops, is similar to a civilian maintenance organization (HMO), where each enrollee is assigned a "gatekeeper" who provides primary care and authorizes referrals for specialty care. Beneficiaries receive care from a Military Treatment Facility (MTF) when available. If services are not available at the MTF, or the enrollee does not live near an MTF, he or she may seek care from a provider in the TRICARE network—a network of civilian health professionals. A point of service option is also available for care received without a referral, but results in higher out-of-pocket costs.

Although the TRICARE benefit covers outpatient mental health, service members who rely on the TRICARE network often have limited access to services. The DoD Task Force on Mental Health found that many providers on the TRICARE network provider list were not accepting TRICARE patients. A recent GAO survey of Reservists, most of whom had prior experience with private insurance coverage, also highlighted the paucity of available TRICARE network providers. Although the survey did not focus on mental health providers specifically, it found that only 12 percent of Reservists felt that the availability of providers and specialists was better in TRICARE than in the private sector, compared to 50 percent who felt that availability was better in the private sector (US GAO Feb 2007).

While there are some areas where TRICARE seems to be providing an accessible continuum of mental health services, this is not generally the case. With increased deployments of National Guard and Reserve members who have time limited TRICARE coverage for themselves and their families, combined with increasing demand for services from families and retirees and the deployment of mental health professionals who would otherwise be providing services on base, the networks are stretched to their limit. TRICARE has difficulty expanding the network because of low reimbursement rates and fragmented rules (US DoD Task Force on Mental Health 2007).

The DoD Mental Health Task Force determined that the TRICARE continuum of care for mental health services is severely deficient. Intensive outpatient care, one of the most frequently utilized services in private and VA care is not covered at all, substance abuse treatment options are limited, characterized by very poor access, and well below the level offered even by Medicaid. Crucial early intervention services including marital/family counseling and early intervention for hazardous substance misuse are not covered (US DoD Task Force on Mental Health 2007).

Based on recommendations from the DoD Mental Health Task Force, the Secretary of Defense has undertaken efforts to increase staffing, increase recruitment and improve the continuum of TRICARE services.

3. Veterans Health Administration

VA operates the nation's largest integrated health care system with over 210,000 employees and a budget of $37.3 billion. In fiscal year 2007, VA provided health care to approximately 5.6 million veterans at 157 VA Medical Centers and 875 community-based outpatient clinics nationwide (US Department of Veterans Affairs 2008). As of April 2007, over one-third (35 percent) of the 717,000 OEF/OIF veterans, who were eligible for VA services, sought VA care, most commonly for musculoskeletal injuries and mental health issues.

VA has undergone significant positive changes in the past 10-15 years. It has become an integrated system that is, by many measures, producing the highest quality care in the country (Longman 2005).

This improvement can be credited at least partially to the system being decentralized, with treatment being shifted to more outpatient settings. The system is now divided into 21 regional "Veterans Integrated Service Networks" that administer health services and tailor service delivery to local needs and conditions. In addition to decentralization, VA also developed an electronic medical record system (VISTA) heralded as a model for other providers (Frist 2005). These significant improvements notwithstanding, VA continues to face challenges in adapting the current health care delivery to meet the unparalleled incidence of PTSD and TBI in the returning OEF/OIF veteran population.

There is concern that VA is not geographically accessible to all veterans. Approximately 39 percent of veterans reside in rural areas. Although according to VA, over 92 percent of enrollees reside within one hour of a VA facility, and 98.5 percent are within 90 minutes, this includes small community based outpatient clinics, which offer very limited or no mental health services (Cross 2007). Some argue that VA should consider itself the healthcare provider for all veterans and provide services both through VA staffed clinics and where necessary, due to travel time or other factors, through contractual arrangements with local providers.

Vet Centers: In addition to the medical centers and clinics, VA has 209 Veterans Readjustment Centers known as "Vet Centers." They have a considerable degree of autonomy and thus can tailor services and staffing to meet the specific cultural and psychological needs of the veterans they serve. Although the centers get some support from VA health centers, they are separate entities and guarantee that anything said at the Vet Center stays at the Vet Center. VA is implementing plans to expand the number of Vet Centers to 232 within the next two years.

Every Vet Center has at least one VA qualified mental health professional on staff. In FY 2006, the Vet Center program had 1,066 assigned staff positions of which 159 were outreach specialists and 876 were authorized counseling staff (58 percent of whom were licensed mental health professionals). Vet Centers are generally small, storefront buildings with four or five staff members, two-thirds of whom are veterans (Batres 2007).

One of the distinguishing features of the Vet Center program is its authority to provide services to veterans' immediate family members. As noted earlier, family participation can be critical to the success of treatment. Therefore, family members are included in the counseling process, to the extent necessary to treat the veterans' readjustment issues. Veterans' immediate family members are also eligible for care at Vet Centers. In addition, Vet Centers offer bereavement counseling to surviving family members.

Outreach for OIF/OEF veterans: VA has invested new resources to reach out to OIF/OEF veterans. Hundreds of outreach workers, mostly OIF/OEF veterans have been hired by both the VA medical centers and Vet Centers. These outreach workers and other VA staff members attend all demobilization activities for National Guard and Reserve Units, and attempt to in general make OIF/OEF veterans aware of services and facilitate their use of services.

Screening and Assessment: VA provides screening for mental health issues, including depression, PTSD, and substance abuse in all primary care clinics. Recently VA implemented universal screening for TBI for all OIF/OEF veterans. Patients screening positive on any of the mental health or TBI screens are further evaluated and triaged to treatment as indicated.

Treatment: VA offers a continuum of care for patients with mental disorders but not all types of care may be available to each client. For PTSD each medical center has at least one therapist who specializes in the care of patients with stress disorders. Most have an interdisciplinary PTSD team, and at selected medical centers intensive outpatient, residential or impatient programming is available. A few medical centers have programs specifically dedicated to female veterans or veterans with comorbid substance abuse. A few of the largest Community Outpatient Clinics offer specialized PTSD care, but most offer only general mental health care, and smaller clinics may offer only primary care.

As noted earlier in this chapter, analyses of the effectiveness of PTSD treatments including the most recent Institute of Medicine report indicate that the treatments with proven efficacy are intensive and time consuming to administer. They require specialized training for staff and the availability of time to provide them to veterans. VA has struggled to translate the results of these effectiveness studies to widespread clinical practice across the system. Efforts are ongoing, and VA has created a special office to try to improve the translation of evidence based approaches, but they are still unavailable in many locations.

Some locations, particularly smaller clinics rely on "telemental" therapy, in which clients receive treatment from a remote mental health professional using video conferencing. While preliminary research clearly has established that a variety of telemental health modalities are feasible, reliable, and satisfactory for general clinical assessments and care, much less is known about the clinical application and general effectiveness of telemental health modalities employed in the assessment or treatment of PTSD (Morland et al. u.d)

Waiting lists and waiting times: VA recently completed an analysis of gaps in mental health care throughout the system. This analysis underscored the reality that access to services is still unacceptably variable across the VA system, despite considerable augmentation of programming in the past few years. In response VA is beginning to fund additional initiatives to fill these gaps. For example in September 2008 VA announced it was adding substance use disorder clinicians to PTSD teams at a cost of $13.3 million per year and that it will provide approximately $17 million per year to establish Intensive Outpatient Substance Use Disorder Programs at 28 additional medical centers, bringing the total number of facilities with these programs to 105.

4. Private Sector

A large percentage of veterans, Guard members, and Reservists rely on TRICARE or private insurance provided by their own, or their spouse's, employer. As a result, many providers treating these service members are not part of the military or VA system, and may not be familiar with the unique needs of the population.

Relative to active duty families, members of the National Guard and Reserves and their families have limited access to military chaplains, family support programs, and all other parts of the military landscape designed to support psychological health. Unfortunately, community providers may not be sufficiently aware of or sufficiently trained to fulfill their needs (US DoD Task Force on Mental Health 2007).

The military service branches and VA have undertaken efforts to disseminate knowledge and best practices to civilian health professionals. For example, the Center for Deployment Psychology at the Uniformed Services University of the Health Sciences developed a two-week intensive training course and a series of seminars, and is planning to reach out to both military and civilian psychologists, psychology interns and residents.

Private insurance does not guarantee access to quality mental health services. The President's New Freedom Commission on Mental Health identified several obstacles that prevent insured consumers from getting appropriate care in the private sector. These obstacles include unfair treatment limitations and cost-sharing requirements placed on mental health benefits, and a fragmented mental health delivery system (President's New Freedom Commission on Mental Health 2003). As the Institute of Medicine points out in *Improving the Quality of Care for Mental and Substance-use Conditions: Quality Chasm Series* (2006), mental health care is frequently delivered in ways that are not consistent with scientific evidence, and often delivered in isolation from general health care, despite the fact that mental illnesses and general health problems are frequently intertwined. Patients receive care from multiple physicians, across multiple sites, and in multiple delivery systems. These different entities often fail to coordinate care or share information. This failure to collaborate jeopardizes patients' health and recovery. Collaboration is especially difficult because mental health substance-use problems are often addressed by public-sector programs apart from private-sector general health care.

5. Nonprofit and Volunteer Organizations

Numerous nonprofit and volunteer organizations provide creative approaches to reducing PTSD symptoms and helping service members and veterans reintegrate into society. These types of programs could play an important role in encouraging veterans to seek longer-term professional care or in supplementing traditional therapies. For example:

- Organizations such as Give an Hour, Operation Comfort, Strategic Outreach to Families of All Reservists (SOFAR), the Colorado Psychological Association, and The Returning Veterans Project NW provide free counseling services.
- The Wounded Warrior Project has a weeklong adventure program including ropes courses, water sports, and a Native American healing ritual.
- The Valley Forge Return to Honor Workshop offers complimentary three-day intensive cognitive and experiential reintegration workshops.
- The Merritt Center offers complimentary retreat programs that include walks in the woods, sweat lodge ceremony, therapeutic massage, release exercises of body and mind and other relaxation strategies.

Some programs serve a small geographic area, while others are nationwide. Each program performs its own outreach based on its available resources. These programs have no national registry.

Section 6. Barriers to Seeking Care

I served in Baghdad from April 2003 to May 2004... September of 2003 I was sent for treatment ...I met with a Major there a couple of times who put me on three different antidepressants. For those of you who have been there, you know how difficult this is. For one, just the PTSD and Combat Stress Control is a huge stigma that generally isn't viewed too kindly by the chain of command. Add to this the fact that I was an NCO in charge of a combat engineer team who prided themselves in their "sapper" skills.

But the other difficult part is actually getting the antidepressants you were prescribed. For us, there wasn't a pharmacy anywhere nearby; you had to go to the Green Zone.

Lejeune, Chris. From his blog on The VetVoice Diaries.

Researchers have found that among the military service members who have returned from Iraq and Afghanistan and report symptoms of post traumatic stress disorder or major depression, only slight more than half have sought treatment (Tanielian and Jaycox 2008). Barriers to seeking care fall into two general categories: stigma and access (Hoge et al. 2004).

1. Stigma

Three unique types of stigma pose barriers to treatment (Sammons 2005):

Public Stigma refers to the public (mis)perceptions of individuals with mental illnesses. Over half of surveyed soldiers who met criteria for a psychological health problem thought they would be perceived as weak, treated differently, or blamed for their problem if they sought help (Hoge et al. 2004; US DoD Task Force on Mental Health 2007).

Self Stigma refers to the individual internalizing the public stigma and feeling weak, ashamed and embarrassed.

Structural Stigma refers to the institutional policies or practices that unnecessarily restrict opportunities because of psychological health. Service members repeatedly report believing that their military careers will suffer if they seek psychological services. They believe that seeking care will lower the confidence of others in their ability, threaten career advancement and security clearances, and possibly cause them to be removed from their unit (US DoD Task Force on Mental Health 2007).

The Army has made a concerted effort to reduce the stigma associated with psychological health issues and the efforts seem to have had a positive effect. Based on the Army's annual survey of soldiers in theater, fewer soldiers who met the screening criteria for a mental disorder report that stigma affected their decision to seek treatment in 2007 than in 2006. However, the levels remain unacceptably high as over half of male soldiers in Iraq who meet the screening criteria were concerned that they "would be seen as weak" and 40 percent believed that their leaders would blame them for the problem (US Army Surgeon General 2008) (Exhibit 4).

2. Access

Even when service members or veterans decide to seek care, they need to find the "right" provider at the "right" time. As described in section 5, this is not always possible. When care is not readily available the "window of opportunity" may be lost.

In contrast to the data collected by DoD on barriers to mental health care, there is currently a dearth of information on barriers to care for OIF/OEF veterans seeking VA care. VA publishes patient satisfaction data, but by definition this data only reflects the views of veterans who have overcome whatever barriers that exist and succeeded in gaining access to care. A feedback loop which includes the systematic collection of data on the perception of consumers about the ease of access to care is crucial to identify and decrease barriers to care. No such mechanism for VA care currently exists.

A recurring survey of a national sample of OIF/OEF veterans, including those who do not currently utilize VA services could identify barriers to care, such as: distance from required specialized services; availability of specified types of service including early intervention services; bureaucratic obstacles to accessing care; user friendliness; clinic hours and policies; perceived stigma and concerns with impact on job or reserve unit status; and lack of information about what services are available.

Exhibit 4. Perceived Barriers to Seeking Mental Health Services, 2006 and 2007

Factors that Affect the Decision to Seek Mental Health Treatment	2006	2007
I would be seen as weak	53	50
Members of my unit might have less confidence in me	51	45
My leaders would blame me for the problem	43	39
It would harm my career	34	29
It would be too embarrassing	37	34

Source: Data from MHAT-V 2008

3. Additional Issues for Certain Populations

A. *Culturally Diverse Populations*

Little attention has been paid to the unique needs of culturally diverse populations with PTSD. Despite high rates of PTSD, African-American, Latino, Asian, and Native American veterans are less likely to use mental health services for several reasons:

Cultural competency of providers: A study of Native American and Latino veterans identified several barriers to VA services: 85 percent felt "VA care-givers know little about ethnic cultures," and 79 percent felt that "VA care-givers have problems talking with ethnic veterans" (Nugent et al. 2000). Although little research on the issue specifically focuses on veterans, studies in the civilian sector suggest that individuals are more likely to follow through with therapy if the clinician and client are matched ethnically (Norris and Alegria 2005). The scarcity of minority providers makes this unlikely for most nonwhite veterans. In addition, many intervention materials are unknowingly embedded with cultural expectations and unsubstantiated assumptions about such issues as time orientation, social and occupational commitments, family structure, and gender roles.

Stigma: Compared to white veterans, African-American veterans are more likely to feel shame and guilt for their PTSD. Latinos are more likely to believe that asking for help will bring dishonor to their families. These responses are exacerbated because both groups are more likely to feel that a health provider has judged them unfairly (Norris and Alegria 2005).

Linguistic access: Although most service members and veterans are fluent in English, their family members may have limited English proficiency. Given the important role of families in encouraging veterans to seek services and in locating those services, multilingual outreach and family support is necessary. VA-wide publications such as "VA Benefits" are available in several languages. However, most material, including outreach material, is developed by local or regional VA entities (such as a Vet Center or a VISN), and those entities develop materials in languages other than English at their discretion. The VA Center for Minority Veterans encourages, but cannot require, that materials be available in other languages.

B. Women

Women make up about 10 percent of the US forces in Iraq and Afghanistan. Some of these women have been returning from Iraq not only with combat-related trauma, but also with Military Sexual Trauma (MST). Although estimates vary, between 13 percent and 30 percent of women veterans experienced rape, and a higher percentage experienced some type of sexual trauma over the course of their military careers. The sexual trauma combined with combat trauma makes women far more likely to experience PTSD (Yeager et al. 2006).

The military's response to individual reports of MST, and the barriers that women face in reporting this trauma, is beyond the scope of this chapter. VA has established a number of programs to address the impact, including Military Sexual Trauma counseling, Women Veterans Stress Disorders Treatment Teams, and MST centers.

Section 7. Family Issues

There is a child in my life who thinks I am a hero, a point which is certainly debatable. He was simply happy that I returned home in one piece—at least he thought I was in one piece—and ready to start our lives over from the point at which we left off. However, it fast became apparent to him that I am not the same person he knew before I left, and he is confused by that. He wants the "old me" back and so do I. It is painful and disappointing for both of us.

An Army Reservist who returned from Iraq and Kuwait. From her blog "Citizen Soldier Sojack in OIF."

Service members return home to various types of support systems that may include parents, spouses, children, and significant others. These support systems are critical to the well-being of the veteran with PTSD and TBI. However, they are particularly at risk because family members often do not have access to psychological and informational support services. Providing these services is particularly important for several reasons:

- Family members are often the first to identify that the veteran is having difficulty, and are often instrumental in motivating the veteran to seek professional services. In addition, family members provide critical social and emotional support for the veteran, and may relieve some stress by taking care of many of the veteran's day-to-day responsibilities (US DoD Task Force on Mental Health 2007, Hirsel 2007).
- PTSD can create a circular momentum where the service member's PTSD increases the stress in the spouse, which puts stress on the relationship, which then intensifies the PTSD symptoms in the soldier.
- The veteran's PTSD impacts the psychological health of other family members and caretakers. This has important implications for the well-being of these individuals, as well as for their ability to support the service member (Galovski and Lyons 2004).

1. Effect of PTSD/TBI on the Family

More than 60 percent of service members are married, and almost 50 percent have children.

For some, returning from deployment is a joyous experience. For others, reintegrating back into the family is difficult. It is not uncommon that at the beginning both the spouse and service member have unrealistic expectations of a rapid return to "normal." Both partners soon realize that the service member is not the same as when that service member left and that the family also has changed—spouses have become more independent and developed new routines, and children have gotten older. New family roles and routines must be negotiated (American Psychological Association 2007).

This situation is more challenging for service members who return home with PTSD or depression. The natural tension is exacerbated by the service member's emotional numbness, their apparent disinterest, their reduced ability to solve problems, and their often violent temper. Studies have shown that veterans with psychological injuries are less sure about their role in the household, and are more likely than others to report feeling like a guest in their own home. Those with PTSD are more likely to report that their children acted afraid, or did not act warmly to them (Sayers 2008).

In some cases parents, spouses, and children display symptoms of PTSD because they are upset by the service member's symptoms—a phenomenon known as *secondary traumatization.*

Children are at risk for *intergenerational transmission of trauma* and addressing the concern can be delicate. For example, research shows the following (Ochberg and Peabody 2008):

- When a family silences a child, or teaches him/her to avoid discussions of events, situations, thoughts, or emotions, the child's anxiety tends to increase. He or she may start to worry about provoking the parent's symptoms. Without understanding the reasons for their parent's symptoms, children may create their own ideas about what the parent experienced, which can be even more horrifying than what actually occurred.
- Overdisclosure can be just as problematic. When children are exposed to graphic details about their parent's traumatic experiences, they can start to experience their own set of PTSD symptoms in response to the horrific images generated.
- Children who live with a traumatized parent may start to identify with the parent and begin to share in his or her symptoms as a way to connect with the parent.
- Children may also be pulled to reenact some aspect of the traumatic experience because the traumatized parent has difficulty separating past experiences from present.

2. Services for Family Members

Despite the challenges that families face, they often have difficulty obtaining mental health services. VA provides support for families only through the Vet Centers described in Section 5. These centers provide some psychological health services and support groups. However, the availability of services varies among the different centers. The VA mental health care system may incorporate marital/family interventions when they are focused on improving relationships and reducing veterans' symptoms, but does not offer services targeted at improving the psychological well being of the spouse and children. Marital counseling or family counseling is not readily accessible at many VA facilities.

DoD provides psychological support for families throughout the deployment cycle through MTFs, TRICARE, and several nonmedical programs. However, access to on-base services is limited. Many mental health professionals and chaplains are deployed at the same time that family members need their services. As a result, family members are often referred to the TRICARE network where it may be difficult to find a therapist who is accepting new patients or who has an available appointment time that is not too far in the future. The Army Task Force on Mental Health found that children had particularly constrained access to clinical treatment services, especially adolescents with substance abuse problems (US Army Surgeon General 2008).

Military bases also have nonmedical support services. The armed services vary in what services they offer and how they overlap and coordinate with on base mental health services. Each unit has a Family Readiness Group (FRG), made up of family members, volunteers, and soldiers, that offers family members access to information and social support.

Military OneSource offers confidential resource and referral services that can be accessed 24-hours per day via telephone, the Internet, and e-mail. OneSource provides confidential family and personal counseling services in local communities across the country, at no cost, for up to six sessions per person per problem.

Paradoxically, although the on-base capacity to support psychological health is reduced during deployment in an effort to devote resources to supporting the health of deployed service members, this reduction contributes to the distress of deployed service members who worry about family members at home who cannot obtain needed assistance. Only 21 percent of soldiers serving in Iraq are satisfied with the type of support the military is providing to their families, and only 22 percent think the Family Readiness Group has helped their family. (US Army Surgeon General 2008).

Section 8. Recommendations

The wars in Iraq and Afghanistan are resulting in injuries that are currently disabling for many, and potentially disabling for still more. They are also putting unprecedented strain on families and relationships, strain that can contribute to the severity of the service member's disability over the course of time. NCD concurs with the recommendations of previous Commissions, Task Forces and national organizations that:

1. A comprehensive continuum of care for mental disorders, including PTSD, and for TBI should be readily accessible by all service members and veterans. This requires adequate staffing and adequate funding of VA and DoD health systems.
2. Mechanisms for screening service members for PTSD and TBI should be continuously improved.
3. The current array of mental health and substance abuse services covered by TRICARE should be expanded and brought in line with other similar health plans

    It is particularly critical that prevention and early intervention services be robust. Effective early intervention can limit the degree of long term disability and is to the benefit of the service member or veteran, his or her family and society. Therefore NCD recommends:
4. Early intervention services such as marital relationship counseling and short term interventions for early hazardous use of alcohol and other substances should be strengthened and universally accessible in VA and TRICARE.

    Consumers play a critical role in improving the rehabilitation process. There are many opportunities for consumers to enhance the services offered to service members and veterans and their families. NCD recommends:
5. DoD and VA should maximize the use of OIF/OEF veterans in rehabilitative roles for which they are qualified including as outreach workers, peer counselors and as members of the professional staff.
6. Consumers should be integrally involved in the development and dissemination of training materials for professionals working with OIF/OEF veterans and service members.
7. Current and potential users of VA, TRICARE and other DoD mental health and TBI services should be periodically surveyed by a competent independent body to assess their perceptions of: a) the barriers to receiving care, including distance, cost, stigma, and availability of information about services offered; and b) the quality, appropriateness to their presenting problems and user-friendliness of the services offered.

8. VA should mandate that an active mental health consumer council be established at every VA medical center, rather than have this be a local option as is currently the case.

9. Congress should mandate a Secretarial level VA Mental Health Advisory Committee and a Secretarial level TBI Advisory Committee with strong representation form consumers and veterans organizations, with a mandate to evaluate and critique VA's efforts to upgrade mental health and TBI services and report their findings to both the Secretary of Veterans Affairs and Congress.

    DoD and VA have initiated a number of improvements but as noted by earlier Commissions and Task Forces, gaps continue to exist.

    It is imperative that these gaps be filled in a timely manner. Early intervention and treatment is critical to the long-term adjustment and recovery of service members and veterans with PTSD and TBI. NCD recommends:

10. Congress and the agencies responsible for the care of OEF/OIF veterans must redouble the sense of urgency to develop and deploy a complete array of prevention, early intervention and rehabilitation services to meet their needs now.

As this chapter indicates, the medical and scientific knowledge needed to comprehensively address PTSD and TBI is incomplete. However, many evidence-based practices do exist. Unfortunately, service members and veterans face a number of barriers in accessing these practices including stigma; inadequate information; insufficient services to support families; limited access to available services, and a shortage of services in some areas. Many studies and commissions have presented detailed recommendations to address these needs. There is an urgent need to implement these recommendations.

Acknowledgment

The National Council on Disability wishes to express its appreciation to Nanette Goodman for her work in researching and drafting this document, and to Richard A. McCormick, PhD., Daniel Mont, PhD., Laura McDonald, and Shelley Carson, PhD, for their comments on earlier versions of the paper.

References

A Soldier's Mind. (2008, May 14). Fort Bliss Center Using "Holistic" Approach To Treat PTSD. Accessed August 15, 2008. http://soldiers mind.com/2008/05/14/fort-bliss-center-using-holistic-approach-to-treat-ptsd/

American Psychiatric Association. (1994). *Diagnostic and Statistical Manual of Mental Disorders, Fourth Edition (DSM-IV)*. Washington, DC: American Psychiatric Publishing, Inc.

American Psychological Association, Presidential Task Force on Military Deployment Services for Youth, Families and Service Members (2007, February). *The Psychological Needs of U.S. Military Service Members and Their Families: A Preliminary Report.*

Anonymous (2006, Nov 30). "PTSD Salad." From the blog *This is Your War II.* Accessed September 15, 2008, http://thisisyourwarii.blogspot.com/2006/11/ptsd-salad.html.

Artman, L. & Duckworth, K. (2007). Accommodating Service Members and Veterans with PTSD, *Job Accommodation Network's Consultants' Corner.* Volume, *03*, Issue 02. Accessed July 28, 2008. http://www.jan.w vu.edu/corner/vol03iss02.htm

Barrett, D. H., Doebbeling, C. C., Schwartz, D. A., Voelker, M. D., Falter, K. H., Woolson, R. F. & Doebbeling, D. N. (2002). Posttraumatic Stress Disorder and Self-Reported Physical Health Status Among U.S. Military Personnel Serving During the Gulf War Period A Population-Based Study. *Psychosomatics, 43*,195–205.

Batres, A. R. (2007). Vet Centers Hearing before the Subcommittee on Health of the Committee on Veterans' Affairs. U.S. House of Representatives, 110th Congress. First Session. July 19, 2007.

Belanger, H. G., Vanderploeg, R. D., Curtiss, G. & Warden, D. L. (2007) Recent Neuroimaging Techniques in Mild Traumatic Brain Injury *The Journal of Neuropsychiatry and Clinical Neurosciences, 19*, 5–20.

Bond, G. R (2004). Supported Employment: Evidence for an Evidence-Based Practice. *Psychiatric Rehabilitation Journal, 27(4)*, 345-60.

Boscarino, J. A. (2005). Post-traumatic stress disorder and mortality among U.S. Army veterans 30 years after military service. *Annals of Epidemiology, 16*, 1-9.

Brailey K., Vasterling J. J., Proctor, S. P., Constans, J. I. & Friedman, M. J. (2007). PTSD symptoms, life events, and unit cohesion in U.S. soldiers:

baseline findings from the neurocognition deployment health study. *J Trauma Stress, 20(4)*, 495-503.

Bray, R. M., Hourani, L. L., Omsted, K. L. R., Witt, M., Brown, J. M., Pemberton, M. R., Marsden, M. E., Marriott, B., Schelffler, S., Vandermaas-Peeler, R., Weimer, B., Calvin, S., Bradshaw, M., Close, K. & Hayden, D. (2006). 2005 Department of Defense Survey of Health Related Behaviors Among Active Duty Military Personnel: A Component of the Defense Lifestyle Assessment Program (DLAP). North Carolina: RTI.

Brewin C. R., Andrews B. & Valentine, J. D. (2000). Meta-analysis of risk factors for posttraumatic stress disorder in trauma exposed adults. *Journal of Consulting and Clinical Psychology, 68*, 748–766.

Brewin, C. (2007). *Posttraumatic Stress Disorder: Malady or Myth?* London: Yale University Press.

Bryant, R. A. (2008). Disentangling Mild Traumatic Brain Injury and Stress Reactions. *New England Journal of Medicine, 358(5)*, 525-527.

Chartier, M. (2007). *Implementing Mindfulness in Residential PTSD Care for Veterans: Pilot Data and Lessons Learned.* Presentation to the International Society of Traumatic Stress Studies. Baltimore, Maryland November 17, 2008.

Citizen Soldier Sojack [pseud.] (2007, Oct 26). "The Realities ofDeployment and Readjustment." From her blog *Citizen Soldier Sojack in OIF.* Accessed September 15, 2008. http://sojack.blogspot.com/2007/10/realities-of-deployment-and.html

Cook, J. A., Lehman, A. F., Drake, R., McFarlane, W. R., Gold, P. B., Leff, H. S., Blyler, C., Toprac, M. G., Razzano, L. A., Burke-Miller, J. K., Blankertz, L., Shafer, M., Pickett-Schenk, S. A. 7 Grey, D. D. (2005) Integration of psychiatric and vocational services: a multisite randomized, controlled trial of supported employment. *Am J Psychiatry, 162*, 1948–1956.

Cross, Gerald M. (2007). Acting Principal Deputy Undersecretary for Health Department of Veterans' Affairs. *Statement presented before the Subcommittee on Health House Committee on Veterans' Affairs.* 110th Cong., sess 1. April 18, 2007.

Davidson, J. R. T., Stein, D. J., Shalev, A. Y. & Yehuda, R. (2004). Posttraumatic Stress Disorder: Acquisition, Recognition, Course, and Treatment. *Journal of Neuropsychiatry and Clinical Neuroscience, 16(2)*, 135-147.

Davidson, L., Chinman, M., Kloos, B., Weingarten, R., Stayner, D. & Tebes, J. K. (1999). Peer Support Among Individuals With Severe Mental Illness: A Review of the Evidence. *Clinical Psychology: Science and Practice, 6(2)*, 165 – 187.

Defense Centers of Excellence for Psychological Health and Traumatic Brain Injury, Accessed January 21, 2009. http://www.dcoe.health.mil/About.aspx

Defense Science Board & Department of Defense (2007). Deployment of Members of the National Guard and Reserve in the Global War on Terrorism. Accessed July 10, 2008. http://www.acq.osd.mil/dsb/reports /2007-11-National_Guard_and_Reserve _in_the_Global_War_on_Terrorism.pdf

English, J. T. (2007). The U.S Department of Veterans Affairs Fiscal Year 2008 Health Budget Testimony to the House Committee on Veterans' Affairs. February 14, 2007.

Frist, William. (2005). Why we must invest in electronic medical records. *San Francisco Chronicle*. July 24.

Galovski, T. & Lyons, J. (2004). Psychological sequelae of combat violence: A review of the impact of PTSD on the veteran's family and possible interventions.
Aggression and Violent Behavior, Volume *9,* Issue 5, August 2004, Pages 477-501.

Greenburg, D. L. & Roy, M. J. (2007). In the Shadow of Iraq: Posttraumatic Stress Disorder in 2007. *Journal of General Internal Medicine, 22*, 888– 889.

HelpGuide.org. (2008). *Post-Traumatic Stress Disorder (PTSD): Symptoms, Help, Treatment.* Accessed January 29, 2008. http://www.helpguide.org/ mental/post_traumatic_stress_disorder_symptoms_treatment.htm

Hirsel, H. L. (2007). The Resiliency and Resources Approach to Pos-Deployment Adjustment of OIF/OEF Veterans. Presentation at the 23rd Annual Meeting of the International Society for Traumatic Stress Studies. November 17, 2007: Baltimore, MD.

Hoge, C. W. (2008, March). Testimony to the House Committee on Veterans Affairs, Washington DC: April 1, 2008.

Hoge, C. W., Castro, C. A., Messer, S. C., McGurk, D., Thomas, J. L., Cotting, D. I. & Koffman, R. L. (2004) Combat Duty in Iraq and Afghanistan, Mental Health Problems, and Barriers to Care. *New England Journal of Medicine, 351(1)*, 13-22.

Hoge, C. W., McGurk, D., Thomas, J. L., Cox, A. L, Engel, C. C. & Castro, C. A. (2008). Mild Traumatic Brain Injury in U.S. Soldiers Returning from Iraq. *New England Journal of Medicine, 358(5)*, 453-463.

Hollifield, M., Sinclair-Lian, N., Warner, T. D. & Hammerschlag, R. (2007) Acupuncture for Posttraumatic Stress Disorder: A Randomized Controlled Pilot Trial. *Journal of Nervous & Mental Disease, 195(6)*, 504-513, June 2007.

Hosek, J., Kavanagh, J. & Miller, L. (2006) How Deployments Affect Service Members. Rand Corporation: Santa Monica, CA.

Institute of Medicine & National Research Council (2007). *PTSD and Military Compensation.* Washington DC: National Academies Press.

Institute of Medicine, Committee on Crossing the Quality Chasm: Adaptation to Mental Health and Addictive Disorders (2006). *Improving the Quality of Health Care for Mental and Substance-Use Conditions: Quality Chasm Series.* Washington DC: National Academies Press.

Iverson, A. C., Fear, N. T., Ehlers, Hacker Hughes, J., Hull, L, Earnshaw, M., Greenberg N., Ronal, R., Wessely, S. & Hotopf, M. (2008). Risk factors for post-traumatic stress disorder among UK Armed Forces personnel. *Psychological Medicine, 38*, 511–522.

Johnson, B. (2005). PTSD: What you need to know. *Military.com—Today in the Military.* http://www.military.com/opinion/0,15202,79791,00.html

Koren, D., Doron, N., Cohen, A., Berman, J., Klein, E. M. Increased PTSD Risk With Combat-Related Injury: A Matched Comparison Study of Injured and Uninjured Soldiers Experiencing the Same Combat Events. *American Journal of Psychiatry, 162*, 276–282.

Lejeune, Chris (2008, March 27). "Antidepressant Use In Iraq." From his blog on *TheVetVoice Diaries.* Accessed September 15, 2008. http://www.vetvoice.com/showDiary.do?diaryId=874

Litz, B. T., Engel, C. C., Bryant, R. A. & Papa, A. (2007). A randomized, controlled proof-of-concept trial of an Internet-based, therapist-assisted self-management treatment for posttraumatic stress disorder. *American Journal of Psychiatry, 164(11)*, 1676-83.

Longman, P. (2007). Best Care Anywhere: Why VA Health Care is Better Than Yours. New America Foundation, PoliPointPress: March 2007.

Martinez, T. E & Burt, M. R. (2006). Impact of Permanent Supportive Housing on the Use of Acute Care Health Services by Homeless Adults. *Psychiatric Services, 57*, 992-999.

Maxfield, B. (2006). Army Demographics: 2006 Army Profile. Accessed March 20, 2008. http://www.2k.Army.mil/downloads/FY06Tri-Fold.pdf

McCarroll, J. E., Ursano, R. J. & Fullerton, C. S. (1995). Symptoms of PTSD following recovery of war dead: 13-15 month follow-up. *American Journal of Psychiatry*, *152*, 939-941.

McGough, B (2006, May). *Inside my Broken Skull*. Accessed February 15, 2008   http://www.broken-skull.com/2006_05_01_insidewramc_archive.html

Milliken, C. S., Auchterlonie, J. L. & Hoge, C. W. (2007) Longitudinal Assessment of Mental Health Problems Among Active and Reserve Component Soldiers Returning From the Iraq War. *JAMA, 298(18)*, 2141-2148.

Morland, L., Greene, C., Ruzek, J. & Godleski, L. (u.d). (2008). PTSD and Telemental Health. National Center for PTSD Fact Sheet. Accessed July 11.
http://www.ncptsd.va.gov/ncmain/ncdocs/fact_shts/fs_telemental_health.html

National Council on Disability (2007). *Empowerment for Americans with Disabilities: Breaking Barriers to Careers and Full Employment*. Accessed July 14, 2008 http://www.ncd.gov/newsroom/publications /2007/pdf/ncd94_Employment_20071001.pdf

National Institute of Neurological Disorders and Stroke (2008). NINDS Traumatic Brain Injury Information Page. Accessed December 15, 2008 http://www.ninds.nih.gov/disorders/tbi/tbi.htm

Norris, F. H. & Alegria, M. (2005). Mental Health Care for Ethnic Minority Individuals and Communities in the Aftermath of Disasters and Mass Violence. *CNS Spectrums—The International Journal of Neuropsychiatric Medicine, 10(2)*, 132-140

Nugent, S., Westermeyer, J. & Canive, J. (2000). Assessing Barriers to Mental Health Care Seeking among American Indian and Hispanic American Veterans in Minnesota and New Mexico. *Abstr Acad Health Serv Res Health Policy Meet.*

O'Bryant, J. & Waterhouse, M. (2006) *U.S. Forces in Iraq*. CRS Report for Congress. Order Code RS22449.

O'Hanlon, M. E. & Campbell, J. H. (2008, December 11). Iraq Index Tracking Variables of Reconstruction & Security in Post-Saddam Iraq. Accessed September 15, 2008 http://www.brookings.edu/saban/iraq-index.aspx

Ochberg, F. & Peabody, C. (2008) Post Traumatic Stress in the Military. in *Your Connection to Military Friendly Businesses, Resources, Benefits, Information and Advice*. Edited by the Military Family Network. Virginia: Capital Books.

Perl, L. (2007, May 31). *Veterans and Homelessness*. Congressional Research Service: Report to Congress. RL 34024.

Presidents New Freedom Commission on Mental Health. (2003). Achieving the Promise: Transforming Mental Health Care in America. Accessed July 14, 2008. http://www.mentalhealthcommission.gov/reports/reports.htm

Riddle, J. R., Smith, T. C., Smith, B., Corbeil, T. E., Engel, C. C., Wells, T. S., Hoge, C. W., Adkins, J., Zamorski, M. & Blazer, D. (2007). Millennium cohort: the 2001–2003 baseline prevalence of mental disorders in the U.S. military. *Journal of Clinical Epidemiology, 60*, 192–201.

Rona R. J., Fear, N. T., Hull, L., Greenberg, N., Earnshaw, M., Hotopf, M. & Wessely, S. (2007). Mental health consequences of overstretch in the UK armed forces: first phase of a cohort study. *BMJ*. 2007 Sep 22, *335(7620)*, 571-2.

Rowan, A. B. & R. L. Campise.(2006). A multisite study of Air Force outpatient behavioral health treatment-seeking patterns and career impact. *Military Medicine, 171*, 1123–1127.

Sammons, M. T. (2005). Psychology in the Public Sector: Addressing the Psychological Effects of Combat in the U.S. Navy. *American Psychologist*. November: 899-909

Sayers, S. (2008, March 11). Hearing on Services to the families of wounded warriors. Committee on Veterans' Affairs, US. Senate.

Scurfield, R. (2006). War Trauma: Lessons Unlearned From Vietnam to Iraq. New York: Algora Publishing.

Smith, M., Schnurr, P. & Rosenheck, R. (2005). Employment Outcomes and PTSD Symptom Severity. *Mental Health Services Research, 7(2)*, 89-101.

Solomon, P. (2004). Peer Support/Peer Provided Services: Underlying Processes, Benefits, and Critical Ingredients. *Psychiatric Rehabilitation Journal, (27)4*, 392-401.

SPC Freeman [pseud.], (2007, April 14) "The Problem of Perception." From his blog The Calm Before the Sand. Accessed September 15, 2008 http://calmbeforethesand.blogspot.com/2007_04_01_archive.html

Stathopoulou, G., Powers, M. B., Berry, A. C., Smits, J. A. J. & Otto, M. W. (2006). Michael W. Otto (2006) Exercise Interventions for Mental Health: A Quantitative and Qualitative Review. *Clinical Psychology: Science and Practice, 13 (2)*, 179–193

Tanielian, T. & Jaycox, L. H. (2008). *Invisible Wounds of War Psychological and Cognitive Injuries, Their Consequences, and Services to Assist Recovery*. Santa Monica, CA: Rand Corporation. Accessed July 1, 2008. http://www.rand.org/pubs/monographs/MG720/

US Army Surgeon General. (2008, February). *Mental Health Advisory Team (MHAT) V: Operation Iraqi Freedom 06-08: Iraq Operation Enduring Freedom 8: Afghanistan.* Accessed July 9, 2008. http://www.Army medicine.Army.mil/reports/mhat/mhat_v/mhat-v.cfm

US Army Walter Reed Army Institute of Research, *Battlemind Training: Continuing the Transition Home.* https://www.battlemind.Army.mil/ assets/files/battlemind_training_ii.ppt#444 Continuing the Transition Home Training Timeframe: 3-6 months post-deployment.

US Army Walter Reed Army Institute of Research, *Battlemind Training: Continuing the Transition Home.* Accessed December 15 https://www.battlemind.army.mil/

US Department of Defense Task Force on Mental Health. (2007). *An achievable vision: Report of the Department of Defense Task Force on Mental Health.* Falls Church, VA: Defense Health Board.

US Department of Labor. (2009). America's Heroes at Work Program. Accessed January 21. http://www.americasheroesatwork.gov/

US Department of Veterans Affairs & Department of Defense (VA/DoD). (2004). *VA/DoD Clinical Practice Guideline for the Management of Post Traumatic Stress.* Accessed July 15, 2008. http://www.guideline.gov /summary/summary.aspx?ss=15&doc_id=5187

US Department of Veterans Affairs & Office of Inspector General. (2007). *Healthcare Inspection Implementing VHA's Mental Health Strategic Plan Initiatives for Suicide Prevention.* Report No. 06-03706-126

US Department of Veterans Affairs & Office of the Inspector General. (2007). Healthcare Inspection: Implementing VHA's Mental Health Strategic Plan Initiatives for Suicide Prevention. Washington DC: VA Office of Inspector General. Accessed March 21, 2008. http://www.va.gov/oig/ 54/reports/VAOIG-06-03706-126.pdf

US Department of Veterans Affairs (2008, February). FY07 VA Information pamphlet. Accessed March 31, 2008. http://www1.va.gov/vetdata /docs/Pamphlet_2-1-08.pdf

US Department of Veterans Affairs (2008, May). Homeless Programs & Initiatives. Accessed July 15, 2008. http://www1.va.gov/homeless /page.cfm?pg=2

US Government Accountability Office (GAO). (2006, Mar). *Military Disability System: Improved Oversight Needed to Ensure Consistent and Timely Outcomes for Reserve and Active Duty.* GAO-06-362

US Government Accountability Office (GAO). (2006, May). *Post-Traumatic Stress Disorder: DoD Needs to Identify the Factors Its Providers Use to*

Make Mental Health Evaluation Referrals for Servicemembers. GAO-06-397

US Government Accountability Office (GAO). (2007, Feb). *Military Health: Increased TRICARE Eligibility for Reservists Presents Educational Challenges.* GAO-07-195

US Government Accountability Office (GAO). (2007, Oct). *Defense Health Care: DoD Needs to Address the Expected Benefits, Costs, and Risks for Its Newly Approved Medical Command Structure.* GAO-08-122

US Government Accountability Office (GAO). (2008, Feb). *VA Health Care: Mild Traumatic Brain Injury Screening and Evaluation Implemented for OEF/OIF Veterans, but Challenges Remain.* GAO-08-276

Veterans Affairs Canada. (2006*). Operational Stress Injury Social Support* (OSISS) Program   Accessed December 15, 2008 http://www.vac-acc.gc.ca/clients/sub.cfm?source=mhealth/osi_prog

Veterans for Common Sense. (2008). *VA Fact Sheet: Impact of Iraq and Afghanistan Wars.* Accessed March 25, 2008. http://veterans.house.gov /Media/File/110/2-7-08/VA-DoDfactsheet.htm

Waterhouse, M. & O'Bryant, J. (2008). National Guard Personnel and Deployments: Fact Sheet. Congressional Research Service: Order code RS22451. Updated January 17, 2008. Accessed July 10, 2008. http://www .fas.org/sgp/crs/natsec/RS22451.pdf

Yeager, D. Himmelfarb, N. Cammack, A. & Mintz, J. (2006) DSM-IV Diagnosed Posttraumatic Stress Disorder in Women Veterans With and Without Military Sexual Trauma. *Journal of General Internal Medicine, 21,* S65–69.

In: Hidden Wounds: Traumatic Brain Injury ...   ISBN: 978-1-61122-415-3
Editor: Joseph R. Phillips   © 2011 Nova Science Publishers, Inc.

Chapter 3

Traumatic Brain Injury: Better DOD and VA Oversight Can Help Ensure More Accurate, Consistent and Timely Decisions for the Traumatic Injury Insurance Program

United States Government Accountability Office

Why GAO Did This Study

More than 1.6 million American service members have deployed to Iraq and Afghanistan in Operation Iraqi Freedom (OIF) and Operation Enduring Freedom (OEF). As of December 2008, more than 4,000 troops have been killed and over 30,000 have returned from a combat zone with visible wounds and a range of permanent disabilities. In addition, an estimated 25-40 percent have less visible wounds—psychological and neurological injuries associated with post traumatic stress disorder (PTSD) or traumatic brain injury (TBI), which have been dubbed "signature injuries" of the Iraq War.

What GAO Recommends

GAO recommends that DOD and VA (1) implement a quality assurance review process to help ensure that decisions are accurate and consistent within and across the services and (2) take steps to ensure the data required to assess the approval rate for traumatic brain injury and timeliness of the claims process are reliable and comprehensive. DOD and VA generally agreed with our recommendations.

What GAO Found

Although VA data show that 63 percent of servicemembers with traumatic brain injury were approved for TSGLI, the actual approval rate may be lower, and DOD and VA lack assurance that claim decisions are accurate, consistent, and timely within and across the branches of service. VA's data show that 520 of the 821 servicemembers who filed TSGLI claims for traumatic brain injury received benefits. However, the actual approval rate may be lower because VA does not include all denials for traumatic brain injury in its data. In addition, DOD and VA officials told us there is no systematic quality assurance review process to ensure that claim decisions are accurate and consistent within and across the services. Finally, DOD and VA lack reliable data on how long it takes the services to make decisions on traumatic brain injury claims.

We identified three major challenges servicemembers with traumatic brain injury have faced and found that DOD and VA have taken a number of steps to address these challenges and expand access to the program. First, while TSGLI is intended as a quick benefit, servicemembers have had difficulties in starting claims soon after their injuries, in part because of a lack of awareness about the program. In response, DOD placed TSGLI staff in 10 of its largest medical treatment facilities to educate servicemembers and help them file claims. Second, the eligibility criteria for traumatic brain injury in place at the time of our review were subjective and unclear, which created some challenges for servicemembers. The criteria stated that a servicemember with traumatic brain injury must be completely dependent on another person to perform two of six activities of daily living, such as eating or getting dressed. However, medical providers may have differing opinions on whether someone who requires verbal instructions or reminders to perform these activities is considered completely dependent. VA has since clarified that a servicemember who requires verbal assistance is eligible, but acknowledged that subjectivity still exists in assessing functional ability. Third, servicemembers with traumatic brain injury have faced challenges in obtaining medical records to prove that they meet eligibility criteria. VA made a change to the program to allow servicemembers who can document a 15-day hospital stay to be eligible for a minimum benefit. DOD and VA are reviewing all claims that were denied or approved for less than the maximum amount to determine whether servicemembers are now eligible under these changes.

Abbreviations

DOD   Department of Defense
OSGLI   Office of Servicemembers' Group Life Insurance
OTI   other traumatic injury
TBI   traumatic brain injury

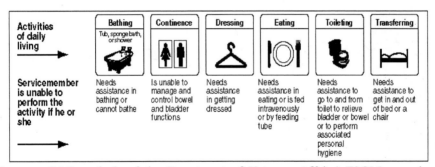

Sources: GAO analysis of the Department of Veterans Affairs' TSGLI procedural guide (August 2007); Art Explosion (images).

TSGLI Activities of Daily Living Eligibility Criteria for Traumatic Brain Injury

TSGLI   Servicemembers' Group Life Insurance Traumatic Injury
Protection

             Program
VA   Department of Veterans Affairs

January 29, 2009

The Honorable Darrell Issa

Ranking Member
Committee on Oversight and Government Reform
House of Representatives

Dear Mr. Issa:

Traumatic brain injury is one of the most common wounds of the current military operations in Afghanistan and Iraq. The nature of these conflicts—in particular, the widespread use of improvised explosive devices—increases the likelihood that servicemembers will be exposed to incidents such as blasts that can cause a traumatic brain injury, which is defined as an injury caused by a blow or jolt to the head or a penetrating head injury that disrupts the normal function of the brain. In 2008, the RAND Corporation estimated that about 20 percent, or 320,000, of U.S. servicemembers returning from Afghanistan and Iraq suffered some type of traumatic brain injury during their deployment.[1]

The number of these and other traumatic injuries suffered by servicemembers in the current conflicts led Congress to create the Servicemembers' Group Life Insurance Traumatic Injury Protection Program, known as TSGLI, in 2005. TSGLI is intended to provide a quick lump sum payment to help address the financial burdens that servicemembers and their families face as a result of their injury. Benefits are intended to meet servicemembers' needs after their injuries but before they start receiving veterans' benefits. For example, the benefits may enable a spouse to leave his or her job and relocate to be with the injured servicemember during treatment and rehabilitation. TSGLI is an insurance benefit attached as a rider to the existing Servicemembers' Group Life Insurance program. The program is modeled after commercial accidental death and dismemberment policies and covers injuries such as loss of hearing or vision or loss of a limb. However, TSGLI differs from many commercial policies in that it is tailored to meet the needs of servicemembers by including injuries such as traumatic brain injury.

TSGLI benefits range from $25,000 to $100,000, depending on the type and nature of the traumatic injury. As of June 2008, the program had awarded more than $285 million to over 4,600 injured servicemembers. The Department of Veterans Affairs (VA) is responsible for administering the TSGLI program, in collaboration with the Department of Defense (DOD), while the individual branches of service are responsible for deciding servicemembers' claims.

Questions have been raised about whether servicemembers with traumatic brain injury have faced challenges in accessing benefits, given that their injuries—which may result in more cognitive than physical impairments—may be more difficult to substantiate than other traumatic injuries, such as amputations. To be eligible for benefits, servicemembers with traumatic brain injury must demonstrate that they were unable to perform two of six activities of daily living, such as bathing or eating, for at least 15 consecutive days because of their injury.

At your request, we reviewed TSGLI as it relates to servicemembers with traumatic brain injury. Specifically, we examined (1) the approval rate of TSGLI claims for traumatic brain injury, and whether DOD and VA have assurance that claims are processed accurately, consistently, and in a timely manner and (2) any challenges servicemembers with traumatic brain injury may have faced in accessing TSGLI benefits, and the extent to which DOD and VA have taken steps to address such challenges.

To develop the information for this chapter, we analyzed data VA gathered from its contractor, the Office of Servicemembers' Group Life Insurance, and the services on the number of claimants and the final disposition and timeliness of their claims since the program's inception. We also reviewed TSGLI enacting legislation, VA and service branch implementing regulations and guidance, and VA's year-one review of the program. We interviewed officials from VA, the Office of Servicemembers' Group Life Insurance, and the services about procedures for verifying their data. In addition, we pulled a random sample of 100 claimants' claim forms from VA's contractor's central database of 8,205 claimants, as of June 30, 2008, to assess the reliability of these data. We found the data were sufficiently reliable to report the total number of claimants and the final disposition of their claims, but we identified a key data limitation for reporting approval rates for traumatic brain injury. We also found the data on the timeliness of some key steps in the claims process to be unreliable. Furthermore, we explored the procedures that VA, its contractor, and the services have in place to ensure accuracy and consistency of decision making.[2] We discussed challenges that servicemembers with traumatic brain injury have faced with DOD and VA officials; service branch TSGLI processing office officials; medical professionals, including officials from the Defense and Veterans Brain Injury Center and the Brain Injury Association of America; and military and veterans' advocacy groups. We also discussed such challenges with servicemembers and some family members in group settings and individual interviews, medical providers, and service branch TSGLI staff at Brooke Army Medical Center, Fort Sam Houston, Texas; National Naval Medical Center, Bethesda, Maryland; Walter Reed Army Medical Center,

Washington, D.C.; and the Polytrauma Rehabilitation Center at the Hunter Holmes McGuire VA Medical Center, Richmond, Virginia. We selected these sites because they represent three of DOD's larger medical treatment facilities for servicemembers with traumatic brain injury and one of VA's four designated traumatic brain injury centers. In addition, we conducted telephone interviews with randomly selected servicemembers with traumatic brain injury who have applied for TSGLI and some of their family members. Furthermore, we reviewed data from a customer satisfaction survey of servicemembers who applied for TSGLI benefits, conducted by VA's contractor, and found these data to be reliable for our purposes. See appendix I for a more detailed description of our scope and methodology.

We conducted this performance audit from January 2008 through January 2009 in accordance with generally accepted government auditing standards. Those standards require that we plan and perform the audit to obtain sufficient, appropriate evidence to provide a reasonable basis for our findings and conclusions based on our audit objectives. We believe that the evidence obtained provides a reasonable basis for our findings and conclusions based on our audit objectives.

Results in Brief

Although VA data show that 63 percent of servicemembers with traumatic brain injury were approved for TSGLI, the actual approval rate may be lower, and DOD and VA lack assurance that claim decisions are accurate, consistent, and timely within and across the services. According to VA data, 520 of the 821 servicemembers claiming a loss due to traumatic brain injury were approved, as of June 2008. However, the actual approval rate may be lower because VA's data do not include all denials for traumatic brain injury. We also found that there is no systematic quality assurance review process to ensure that claim decisions are accurate and consistent within and across the services, a key internal control activity and a component of other VA benefits programs. In addition, DOD and VA lack reliable, sufficient data for overseeing TSGLI claims. VA's central database does not capture all key aspects of the claims process, such as the time that it takes the services to make a decision on a claim. VA officials recognized this limitation and began collecting separate timeliness data from the services on a regular basis in 2007. However, the data they have collected since then are unreliable. For example, about one-third of the data on claim processing times that VA provided to us had dates that were missing or out of sequence. Furthermore, the data VA collects from the services do not break out claims by injury. As a result, DOD and VA lack information on how long it takes the services to make decisions on traumatic brain injury claims.

We identified three major challenges that servicemembers with traumatic brain injury have faced—initiating claims, proving that they met eligibility criteria, and providing adequate documentation to support their claims—and DOD and VA have taken a number of steps to address these challenges and expand access to the program for more servicemembers with traumatic brain injury. First, while TSGLI is intended as a quick benefit, servicemembers, including those with traumatic brain injury, have had difficulties in starting claims soon after their injuries. For example, some servicemembers we interviewed reported that they did not apply immediately due to the severity of their injuries or a lack of awareness of the program. In response, DOD placed TSGLI staff in 10 of its largest medical treatment facilities to educate servicemembers about the program and help them navigate the claims process. Second, the eligibility criteria in place at the time of our review for loss of activities of daily living were subjective and unclear, which created challenges for servicemembers with traumatic brain injury in proving that they met the criteria. For example, the criteria stated that a servicemember with traumatic brain injury must be completely dependent on another person to qualify for benefits. However, medical providers may have differing opinions on whether a servicemember with a traumatic brain injury who requires verbal assistance to perform the activities of daily living, such as instructions on how to dress, is considered completely dependent. During the course of our review, VA completed a comprehensive year-one review of the TSGLI program and made changes to the TSGLI claim form and guidance to clarify that a servicemember who requires verbal assistance is eligible. Third, servicemembers with traumatic brain injury have faced challenges in proving they met the eligibility criteria because they lacked medical documentation with sufficient information on the length of time they were unable to perform activities of daily living. To remedy this problem, VA made a change to the program to allow servicemembers who can document a 15-day hospital stay to be eligible for the minimum benefit of $25,000. This change will expand access to the program for more servicemembers with traumatic brain injury as well as those with other traumatic injuries. DOD and VA officials told us they are reviewing all claims that were denied or approved for less than the maximum amount to determine whether the servicemembers are now eligible for an initial or higher TSGLI payment under the clarified guidance for the activities of daily living criteria and the new 15-day hospital stay criterion.

We are making two recommendations to improve management of the TSGLI program and provide greater assurance that injured servicemembers receive accurate, consistent, and timely treatment. We are recommending that the Secretary of Veterans Affairs work with the Secretary of Defense and the branches of service to implement a systematic quality assurance review process to help ensure that TSGLI benefit decisions are accurate and consistent within and across the services. We are also recommending that the agencies work together to take steps to ensure that the data required to assess approval rates for traumatic brain injury and the timeliness of key steps in the TSGLI claims process are reliable and comprehensive.

We provided a draft of this chapter to the Department of Defense; the Department of Veterans Affairs; and VA's contractor, the Office of Servicemembers' Group Life Insurance. DOD and VA provided written comments, shown in appendixes II and III, respectively, and VA also provided technical comments, that we have incorporated into the report as appropriate. The Office of Servicemembers' Group Life Insurance provided oral comments, and we have incorporated them into the report as appropriate. The agencies and the Office of Servicemembers' Group Life Insurance generally agreed with our recommendations.

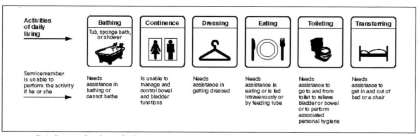

Sources: GAO analysis of the Department of Veterans Affairs' TSGLI procedural guide (August 2007); Art Explosion (images).

Figure 1. Description of Activities of Daily Living Criteria for TSGLI

Background

Traumatic brain injury can vary greatly in terms of severity—from mild cases that might involve a brief change in mental status, such as being dazed or confused, to severe cases that may involve an extended period of unconsciousness or amnesia after the injury. The Defense and Veterans Brain Injury Center classifies brain injuries as mild, moderate, or severe based on factors associated with the initial injury, such as the length of time in a coma, rather than on the symptoms or long-term effects. Servicemembers who sustain even a mild traumatic brain injury may experience short-term physical symptoms such as headaches or dizziness, emotional symptoms such as anxiety or irritability, or cognitive impairments such as difficulty concentrating or sleep disturbances. According to the Defense and Veterans Brain Injury Center, civilian research on brain injury shows that the majority of people with mild traumatic brain injury recover within a few months or a year, but some may experience symptoms related to mild traumatic brain injury months or even years after their injury.[3] Servicemembers also may have other physical injuries in addition to a traumatic brain injury or may suffer from the cumulative effects of multiple blasts that can slow or complicate their recovery. Furthermore, some of the symptoms of mild traumatic brain injury—such as irritability and insomnia—are similar to those associated with other conditions, such as post-traumatic stress disorder.

Although understanding of traumatic brain injury has increased among the medical community in recent decades, according to a DOD task force on traumatic brain injury, gaps remain in research on the short- and long-term effects of traumatic brain injury. DOD is currently investing $300 million in more than 170 research grants to study traumatic brain injury and post-traumatic stress disorder. According to DOD, funds will be used to improve the prevention and treatment of traumatic brain injury and improve the quality of life for people suffering from traumatic brain injury.

While the medical community has established mild, moderate, and severe classifications based on the initial characteristics of traumatic brain injuries, the legislation creating the TSGLI program did not base eligibility on these classifications.[4] Rather, it based eligibility on brain injuries that result in a loss of functioning, specifically the ability to perform two of six activities of daily living. According to VA, the activities of daily living criteria are used by some commercial insurance industry carriers in their disability and long-term care policies. The activities of daily living are (1) bathing, (2) continence, (3) dressing, (4) eating, (5) toileting, and (6) transferring in and out of bed or a chair. See figure 1 for a description of these activities.

In May 2005, Congress created the TSGLI program to provide lump sum payments to traumatically injured servicemembers. According to VA, these payments are intended to provide a short-term benefit during a servicemember's recovery period, whereas the VA disability compensation program is designed to meet the long-term financial needs of servicemembers who lose income-earning potential due to their injuries. The law mandated coverage of certain specific losses, including coma or the inability to perform two of the activities of daily living resulting from traumatic injury to the brain. The law also gave VA the authority to prescribe additional injuries not specifically listed in the law. VA included additional losses by creating an "other traumatic injury" category to cover traumatic injuries that were not specified in the statute. For example, a gunshot wound to the torso could result in multiple injuries that, while not specifically listed in the law, are significant. As with traumatic brain injury, a servicemember must be unable to perform two of six activities of daily living to qualify for benefits under the other traumatic injury category. However, where servicemembers with traumatic brain injury must be unable to perform activities of daily living for at least 15 days to receive a TSGLI benefit, the minimum threshold for servicemembers applying under the other traumatic injury category is 30 days.

Servicemembers who are injured on or after December 1, 2005, the effective date of the program, are eligible to file a claim for a traumatic injury sustained anywhere.[5] Servicemembers injured in a combat zone prior to this date but on or after October 7, 2001—the date military operations in Afghanistan began—are eligible to file a retroactive claim.[6] In 2008, legislation passed the Senate that included a provision that would eliminate the requirement that the traumatic injury be incurred in a combat zone to be eligible for retroactive benefits. That provision was not included in the bill passed by the House of Representatives in September 2008. The Congressional Budget Office estimated that expanding retroactive criteria would make an estimated 700 servicemembers eligible for benefits totaling $47 million.

To qualify for a TSGLI payment:

1. The servicemember's qualifying injury or loss[7] must be directly caused by a traumatic event.
2. The traumatic event must occur before midnight on the day that the member separates from the uniformed services.
3. The servicemember's qualifying injury or loss must occur within 730 days (2 years) of the traumatic event.
4. The servicemember must survive for at least 7 days from the date of the traumatic injury.[8]

5. The injury cannot be caused by a mental disorder, mental or physical illness or disease, among other exceptions.[9]

TSGLI provides payments ranging from $25,000 to $100,000, depending on the type and nature of the injury. Servicemembers may be eligible to be paid for injuries under two or more categories, but they may not receive more than a total of $100,000 for injuries resulting from one traumatic event.[10] See table 1 for the losses covered by TSGLI at the time of our review.

Table 1. TSGLI Schedule of Losses

Qualifying losses	TSGLI benefits
Amputation (loss of foot, hand, or thumb and index finger on the same hand)	$50,000 (or $100,000 for both feet or hands)
Total and permanent loss of speech	$50,000
Total and permanent loss of sight in one eye	$50,000 (or $100,000 for both eyes)
Total and permanent loss of hearing in one ear	$25,000 (or $100,000 for both ears)
Paralysis (quadriplegia, paraplegia, and hemiplegia)	$100,000
Burns (third-degree burn to at least 30 percent of face or 30 percent of body)	$100,000
Coma (for at least 15, 30, 60, or 90 days)	$25,000 for 15 consecutive days up to $100,000 for 90 days
Traumatic brain injury resulting in loss of activities of daily living (for at least 15, 30, 60, or 90 days)	$25,000 for 15 days up to $100,000 for 90 days
Other traumatic injuries resulting in loss of activities of daily living (for at least 30, 60, 90, or 120 days)	$25,000 for 30 days up to $100,000 for 120 days

Source: GAO analysis of the Department of Veterans Affairs' TSGLI procedural guide (August 2007).

Note: On November 26, 2008, VA published interim final regulations that modified the schedule of losses. Among other changes, VA added a $25,000 TSGLI benefit for a 15-day continuous hospital stay due to traumatic brain injury or other traumatic injuries.

VA's Insurance Service is responsible for administering the TSGLI program, setting policies and issuing regulations, in collaboration with DOD.[11] According to agency officials, one way that DOD and VA regularly coordinate is through monthly conference calls to discuss issues related to program administration.[12] VA is responsible for ensuring the financial health of the program, and DOD collects TSGLI premiums—currently $1 per month for servicemembers with full-time coverage through the Servicemembers' Group

Life Insurance program—and forwards them monthly to VA for transfer to the Office of Servicemembers' Group Life Insurance. DOD, through the branches of service, is responsible for covering costs that exceed premium income due to the extra hazards of military service. The services are responsible for developing and deciding servicemembers' claims as well as overseeing reconsiderations and appeals.

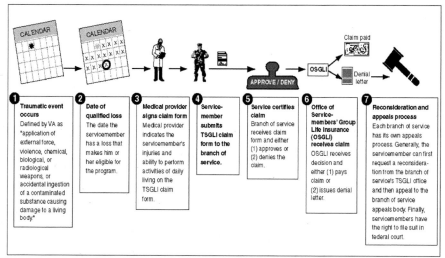

Sources: GAO analysis of the Department of Veterans Affairs' TSGLI procedural guide (August 2007); Art Explosion (images).

Figure 2. Key Steps in the TSGLI Claims Process

The Office of Servicemembers' Group Life Insurance—an office established by a contractor, the commercial life insurance company Prudential—is responsible for paying benefits to servicemembers who are approved and for issuing denial letters to those who are not approved. The Office of Servicemembers' Group Life Insurance is also responsible for centrally recording data on all TSGLI claims, including reconsiderations and appeals. If a servicemember is not satisfied with the decision, he or she may submit additional medical documentation and request that the claim be reconsidered by the TSGLI office within their branch of service. If still not satisfied with the results of the reconsideration, the servicemember can appeal the decision to a branch of service appeals body. See figure 2 for an illustration of the key steps in the TSGLI claims process.

Traumatic Brain Injury Approval Rates May Be Lower Than 63 Percent, and DOD and VA Lack Assurance That TSGLI Decisions Are Accurate, Consistent, and Timely within and across the Services

Although VA data show that 63 percent of servicemembers claiming a traumatic brain injury were approved for TSGLI, the actual approval rate may be lower; and DOD and VA lack assurance that claim decisions are accurate, consistent, and timely within and across the services. The actual approval rate for traumatic brain injury claimants may be lower because VA's data do not include all traumatic brain injury denials. In addition, neither DOD nor VA has a systematic quality assurance review process to ensure that claim decisions are accurate and consistent within and across the services, a key internal control activity and a component of other VA benefits programs. Finally, DOD and VA lack reliable, sufficient data on the timeliness of key steps in the claims process, particularly data on how long servicemembers with traumatic brain injury wait for their benefits after they submit their TSGLI applications.

VA Data Show 63 Percent of Servicemembers Claiming a Traumatic Brain Injury Were Approved, but the Actual Approval Rate May Be Lower

VA's data show that 63 percent of servicemembers who filed a TSGLI claim for traumatic brain injury were approved, but the actual approval rate may be lower because of the way that VA tracks its data. According to VA's data, 821 servicemembers applied for TSGLI benefits for a loss due to traumatic brain injury and 520 (63 percent) were approved, which is higher than the overall TSGLI approval rate of 56 percent. However, these data do not include all traumatic brain injury denials and, as a result, the actual approval rate may be lower.

Officials from VA and the contractor that administers the program—the Office of Servicemembers' Group Life Insurance—told us that they do not include traumatic brain injury claims where, according to the medical provider who signed the claim form, the servicemember did not suffer a loss in his or her ability to perform activities of daily living due to traumatic brain injury.

Officials explained that they do not include these claims in their data due to a software limitation—their system will not allow claims to be recorded in the traumatic brain injury category unless the medical provider indicated a loss in at least one of the six activities of daily living. To record these denied claims, VA places them in the other traumatic injury category. We were unable to determine how many denials were not included in the traumatic brain injury category in VA's data, but we found 4 such denials in our random sample of 100 claims.[13] See figure 3 for an illustration of traumatic brain injury claims that were not included in VA's data.

Finally, the approval rates in VA's data reflect final approval rates because they also include claimants who were initially denied, but who were approved on reconsideration or appeal.[14] If a servicemember is dissatisfied with the initial decision, he or she can request a reconsideration—a review of the denial or request for a higher benefit award based on new medical documentation—or an appeal. About 40 percent of the requests for a review of the initial decision were eventually approved or awarded a higher amount.

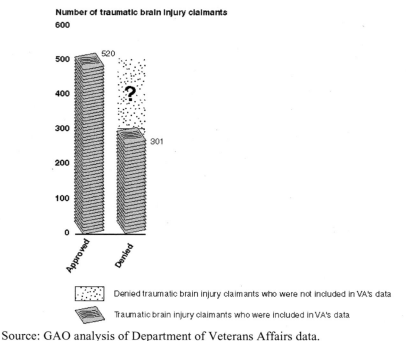

Source: GAO analysis of Department of Veterans Affairs data.

Figure 3. Traumatic Brain Injury Claims Not Included in VA's Approval Rate Data

However, VA could not provide much detail on why claims for traumatic brain injury were denied or why decisions were changed upon reconsideration or appeal. Adjudicators in the services describe why they are denying a claim on the claim form, but VA's contractor groups these reasons into broad categories in VA's data system, such as "provisions not met." As a result, VA has little information across the services on the specific reasons that claims were denied.[15] VA's data also only has a few broad categories to capture the reasons that initial decisions were upheld or reversed. VA officials told us they are improving the level of detail their data will include on the reasons that claims are denied.

DOD and VA Lack Assurance That TSGLI Decisions Are Accurate and Consistent within and across the Services

Neither DOD nor VA has a systematic quality assurance review process to ensure that claim decisions are accurate and consistent within and across the services. A quality assurance review process is a key internal control activity to ensure proper stewardship of federal resources and a component of other VA benefits programs.[16] For example, VA has a quality assurance review process for its disability compensation program, known as the Systematic Technical Accuracy Review, where VA selects random samples of each of its regional offices' decisions and assesses their accuracy in processing and deciding such cases. For the TSGLI program, claim forms should be reviewed by at least two staff members within a service's adjudication office, and VA's contractor, the Office of Servicemembers' Group Life Insurance, performs some checks on the claims before paying them. According to the Office of Servicemembers' Group Life Insurance, claims examiners check claims for obvious errors but do not review medical documentation to determine the accuracy of the services' decisions. In addition, 25 percent of claims are selected for an additional check, which involves verifying information such as a servicemember's name, bank account number, and payment amount.[17] These checks have identified some errors, according to VA officials. For example, one servicemember with traumatic brain injury was initially approved by the branch of service and told he would receive a benefit. However, upon receiving the approved claim form, VA's contractor informed the service that the claim should have been denied because his injury occurred in a non-combat zone 5 months prior to the effective date of the program. The service corrected the error and informed the servicemember that he was not eligible for the program. While these checks have identified some errors, they do not systematically examine whether the services' decisions were correct, nor do they assess consistency within or across the services.

In addition, VA officials noted that the TSGLI approval rates varied across the services, but VA lacked sufficient information to explain these differences. VA officials attributed the Marine Corps' higher overall TSGLI approval rate—67 percent compared with Army's 53 percent approval rate—to the Marine Corps' use of TSGLI staff in medical treatment facilities to assist servicemembers in filing their claims. However, without a quality assurance review process, DOD and VA cannot determine whether differences in approval rates were due to these staff members or to other factors.[18]

Furthermore, while TSGLI allows servicemembers to request a reconsideration or appeal, such a process may not identify whether initial claim decisions were accurate or consistent across the services for two reasons. First, not all servicemembers whose claims are denied will request a claim review. Second, neither DOD nor VA use this process to determine whether original decisions were accurate and consistent across the program, because TSGLI officials from the services told us they allow multiple reconsiderations where servicemembers may submit new medical documentation to support their claim.

During our review, VA officials told us that they planned to review a sample of claim decisions and thought they could build an ongoing, systematic quality assurance process out of this review. Officials told us that, based on what they find, they could send out guidance or make recommendations to the services to improve the accuracy and consistency of TSGLI claim decisions. However, VA had not yet performed such a review.

DOD and VA Lack Reliable, Sufficient Data to Oversee the Timeliness of the Claims Process

DOD and VA lack reliable, sufficient data for overseeing the timeliness of the TSGLI claims process for servicemembers with traumatic brain injury, an important tool in monitoring program performance.[19] VA officials told us that they initially relied on data collected by their contractor, but they recognized that these data do not include all key aspects of the claim process, such as how long the services take to make decisions on servicemembers' claims. As a result, VA requested that the services begin collecting and reporting timeliness data to VA monthly in the spring of 2007. However, we found these data to be unreliable. VA officials acknowledged that there were some problems with the data and stated that about one-third of the data they collected from the services on claim processing times had dates missing or out of sequence. For example, the date the servicemember signed the claim form was prior to the date recorded for the traumatic event that caused the servicemember's injury. Additionally, neither DOD nor VA can assess whether claims for specific injuries take longer than others to process because the data the services send to VA do not break out claims by injury. VA and TSGLI service branch officials stated that the services are generally able to process claims for amputations faster than claims for traumatic brain injury, which involves an assessment of a servicemember's ability to perform activities of daily living; however, there are no data to support this observation.

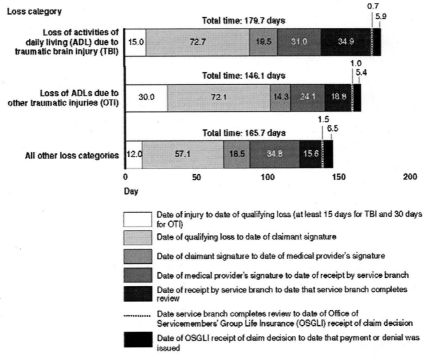

Source: Department of Veterans Affairs, *Servicemembers' Group Life Insurance Traumatic Injury Protection: Year One Review* (July 2008).

Figure 4. VA Study on Average Timeliness of Key Steps in the Claims Process from December 1, 2005, to December 31, 2006

Although VA lacks ongoing and reliable timeliness data, the agency provided us with a reliable, point-in-time study of how many days it took to process 238 claims from December 1, 2005, to December 31, 2006. The sample showed that the services took, on average, 35 days to review and make a decision on traumatic brain injury claims, compared with their goal of processing claims within 30 days. During our review, TSGLI officials from each service stated that their average processing time was less than 30 days; however, VA does not have current, reliable data to support this time frame.

VA's study of the first year of the TSGLI program showed that it took about 180 days from the date a servicemember suffered a traumatic brain injury to the date he or she received a benefit or denial letter. As figure 4 shows, the time it took the services to process servicemembers' claims represented only a small part of this overall time. More than half of this 6-month period elapsed before the services received servicemembers' claims.

Servicemembers with Traumatic Brain Injury Have Faced Challenges in Initiating Claims and Proving Eligibility for TSGLI Benefits, and DOD and VA Have Taken Steps to Address These Challenges

Servicemembers with traumatic brain injury have faced three major challenges to accessing TSGLI benefits—initiating claims, proving that they met eligibility criteria, and providing adequate documentation to support their claims—and DOD and VA have taken a number of steps to address these challenges. For example, DOD has placed TSGLI staff into major medical facilities to assist servicemembers with initiating and filing their claims.

Servicemembers Have Faced Difficulties in Initiating Claims, and DOD Has Placed TSGLI Staff in Major Medical Facilities to Assist Them

Although TSGLI benefits are intended as a quick, short-term benefit, servicemembers with traumatic injuries, including traumatic brain injury, have faced difficulties in initiating claims soon after their injuries. Servicemembers and TSGLI staff that we interviewed told us that support from family immediately after a traumatic injury is important for recovery, and that benefits may enable family members to leave their jobs and relocate to stay with the servicemember during his or her treatment or rehabilitation. For example, one servicemember we interviewed told us that the money he received from TSGLI allowed his family to travel with him to three different hospitals, while another servicemember stated that the money helped his mother, who did not work for 3 months to stay with him during recovery. However, within the first year of the TSGLI program, VA estimated it took servicemembers with traumatic brain injury an average of nearly 3 months to initiate a TSGLI claim. Based on interviews we conducted with servicemembers with traumatic brain injury who applied for TSGLI benefits, the time it took after their injury to initiate a claim ranged from 1 week to 11 months.

Servicemembers with traumatic brain injury have experienced three primary difficulties in initiating TSGLI claims, according to VA and service branch TSGLI officials and servicemembers we interviewed. While there may be other reasons servicemembers waited to apply, many servicemembers did not initiate claims soon after their injuries due to the nature and severity of their traumatic injuries, a lack of awareness of the program, and a lack of assistance in filing the claim.[20] For example:

- Many servicemembers with traumatic brain injury have had multiple severe injuries, and they and their families may have initially focused on treatment and recovery, rather than on benefits. For example, one servicemember we interviewed with a traumatic brain injury told us he did not apply for a TSGLI benefit until more than 2 months after his injury occurred because he was focusing on treating his other injuries—burns to both of his arms.

- Many servicemembers with traumatic brain injury and their families were not aware of TSGLI benefits immediately after the servicemember was injured. One servicemember we interviewed suffered a traumatic brain injury and was in a coma for 3 months due to an automobile accident while on duty in the United States. He spent nearly 8 months in three civilian hospitals and told us he was not aware of the TSGLI program. However, once the servicemember arrived at a VA Medical Center, he told us a TSGLI staff member recognized he would be eligible for benefits and helped him collect medical records from civilian medical providers to support his claim.

Many servicemembers learned about TSGLI a month or more after their injury, according to a 2007 VA survey, and often through informal channels like friends or fellow servicemembers.

- Many servicemembers did not have assistance in gathering medical documentation and filling out the claim form. For example, one servicemember in the National Guard who was taken to a civilian hospital after a car accident in 2007 told us she did not receive assistance in filing her claim and that she had difficulty in gathering medical documentation for the claim. More than half of the servicemembers in VA's survey did not receive assistance in filing their TSGLI claims. In addition, many of the servicemembers we interviewed, especially those who filed claims for injuries incurred close or prior to the implementation of the program in 2005, did not receive any assistance in initiating their claims.

DOD has recognized that servicemembers have faced difficulties in initiating TSGLI claims and has placed TSGLI staff in major medical treatment facilities to help raise awareness about the program and help servicemembers navigate the claims process. One major medical treatment facility—National Naval Medical Center in Bethesda, Maryland—has had in-house Navy and Marine Corps TSGLI staff since early in the program to help servicemembers. TSGLI specialists explain the program's eligibility criteria, assist servicemembers with traumatic injuries in putting together TSGLI claim packets, and act as advocates for the servicemembers. Although they have not conducted a systematic evaluation, DOD and VA officials have partly attributed the Navy's and Marine Corps' higher TSGLI approval rates to this model and recommended expanding it to other treatment facilities. As a result, DOD has placed TSGLI staff in 10 of its largest medical treatment facilities— such as Brooke Army Medical Center at Fort Sam Houston in Texas and Walter Reed Army Medical Center in Washington, D.C.—to help additional servicemembers navigate the claims process. Several of the servicemembers we interviewed benefited from the assistance TSGLI staff members provided. For example, the wife of one servicemember who suffered a traumatic brain injury and several other injuries in Iraq was unaware that her husband was eligible but told us a TSGLI staff member came to her husband's hospital room to inform them about the program and helped them apply for TSGLI.

Some servicemembers with traumatic brain injury are not treated at these major medical treatment facilities and may not benefit from the placement of TSGLI staff, but DOD and VA have proposed steps to provide better outreach to these servicemembers. An Army official told us that servicemembers are increasingly being treated at smaller hospitals, including nonmilitary hospitals, and he has requested additional TSGLI staff to expand their outreach. In addition, during our review, VA completed a comprehensive year-one review of the TSGLI program and proposed several steps to better reach out to servicemembers who may be eligible for the program. For example, VA is exploring using military and VA injury tracking data to periodically identify and notify servicemembers whose injuries may make them eligible for a TSGLI benefit. In addition, VA recently drafted a communications plan, which includes steps such as developing Web-based training and a video on TSGLI as well as revising materials for servicemembers making the transition from military to civilian life and for military and VA staff who assist them.

Servicemembers with Traumatic Brain Injury Have Faced Challenges in Proving Their Eligibility for TSGLI, and VA Has Revised Guidance and Criteria to Improve Access to the Program

Servicemembers with traumatic brain injury have faced challenges in proving they met eligibility requirements, because the criteria in place at the time of our review for loss of activities of daily living were subjective and unclear. For a servicemember to qualify for TSGLI with a traumatic brain injury, a medical provider had to certify that the servicemember was completely dependent on another person to perform at least two of the six activities of daily living for at least 15 days. However, these criteria were subject to interpretation by different medical providers because complete dependency on another person was not clearly defined within the TSGLI claim form. For example, medical providers told us that there may be differing opinions on whether servicemembers with traumatic brain injury who require verbal instructions to dress themselves are completely dependent on another person to perform this activity. Some staff at medical treatment facilities told us that medical providers at their facility would only sign claim forms for loss of activities of daily living if a servicemember was physically dependent on another person. In its year-one review of the TSGLI program, VA acknowledged that the existing guidance on applying the activities of daily living criteria was complicated and subject to different interpretations. As a result, claim decisions could have been inconsistent within and across the services.

In fall 2008, VA revised the TSGLI claim form and guidance to clarify the criteria for loss of activities of daily living. The form and revised guidance clarify that a servicemember is unable to independently perform an activity of daily living if he or she requires either physical assistance, stand-by assistance,[21] or verbal assistance due to a cognitive impairment. See figure 5 for a comparison of the revised claim form and the form in use at the time of our review. Some of the servicemembers we interviewed may now be eligible for benefits with the change in criteria to include stand-by and verbal assistance. For example, one servicemember we interviewed who had a skull fracture and shrapnel in his back from a blast injury in Iraq in 2004 was denied benefits because the service determined he was physically able to perform all of the activities of daily living, despite issues such as nausea and dizziness. However, according to medical documentation, the servicemember is housebound and requires significant assistance from his spouse to perform some activities, such as bathing.

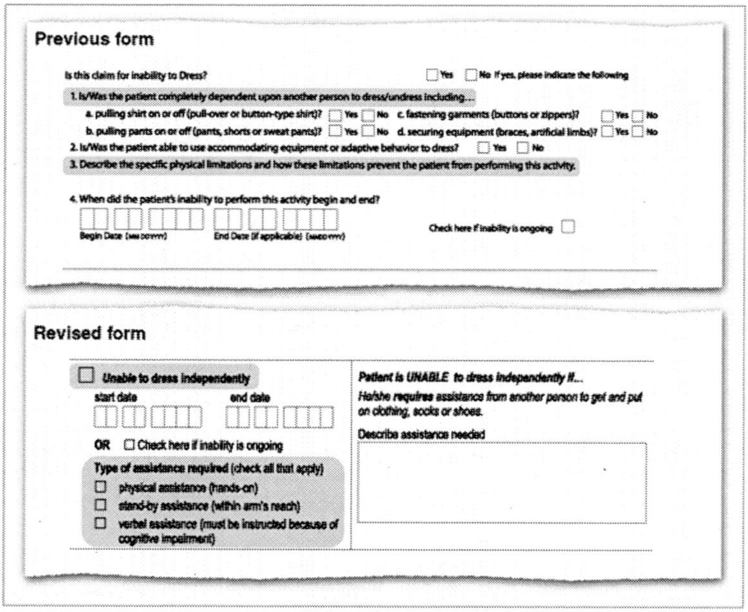

Previous form

Is this claim for inability to Dress? ☐ Yes ☐ No If yes, please indicate the following

1. Is/Was the patient completely dependent upon another person to dress/undress including...
   - a. pulling shirt on or off (pull-over or button-type shirt)? ☐ Yes ☐ No
   - b. pulling pants on or off (pants, shorts or sweat pants)? ☐ Yes ☐ No
   - c. fastening garments (buttons or zippers)? ☐ Yes ☐ No
   - d. securing equipment (braces, artificial limbs)? ☐ Yes ☐ No
2. Is/Was the patient able to use accommodating equipment or adaptive behavior to dress? ☐ Yes ☐ No
3. Describe the specific physical limitations and how these limitations prevent the patient from performing this activity.
4. When did the patient's inability to perform this activity begin and end?

Begin Date (MMDDYYYY) End Date (if applicable) (MMDDYYYY) Check here if inability is ongoing ☐

Revised form

☐ *Unable to dress independently*

start date end date

OR ☐ Check here if inability is ongoing

Type of assistance required (check all that apply)
- ☐ physical assistance (hands-on)
- ☐ stand-by assistance (within arm's reach)
- ☐ verbal assistance (must be instructed because of cognitive impairment)

Patient is UNABLE to dress independently if...

He/she requires assistance from another person to get and put on clothing, socks or shoes.

Describe assistance needed

Sources: Department of Veterans Affairs, Application for TSGLI Benefits (September 2006 and October 2008).

Figure 5. Comparison of the Previous and Revised TSGLI Claim Forms for One Activity of Daily Living

While this revision to the TSGLI claim form and guidance will help clarify the eligibility criteria, VA acknowledged that there are still inherent difficulties in assessing servicemembers' ability to perform activities of daily living. According to medical providers we interviewed, assessing whether servicemembers can perform activities of daily living still involves some subjectivity and professional judgment. However, medical providers told us that the criteria of loss of activities of daily living may be the best available measure for TSGLI benefits because the medical community has not established one objective test to measure a loss of functioning due to traumatic brain injury that could substitute for the current criteria.

According to medical providers we interviewed, traumatic brain injury is diagnosed through multiple assessment tools that are subjective in nature, and these tools cannot easily quantify a loss in cognitive functioning because the loss varies on the basis of the individual and the context of the injury. One such assessment tool, a brain scan, may indicate the area of the brain that is damaged but may not correlate to the actual loss of cognitive functioning. For example, a servicemember we interviewed with 35 years of military service sustained a blast injury in Iraq in December 2006 that resulted in a concussion, and a brain scan indicated damage to more than 60 percent of his brain. However, he continued to perform his duties until he was advised to seek medical attention because fellow servicemembers noticed a change in his behavior. As a result of his traumatic brain injury, the servicemember has been in treatment for over 2 years and continues to have symptoms, such as difficulty in speaking and an inability to sequence steps of a process. He is unable to drive and has gotten lost in his own neighborhood. However, he was able to perform the activities of daily living and did not qualify for TSGLI.

Servicemembers with Traumatic Brain Injury Have Lacked Adequate Medical Documentation for Their TSGLI Claims, but VA Has Established an Alternative to Address This Issue

Servicemembers with traumatic brain injury have faced challenges in proving they met eligibility criteria because they lacked medical documentation with sufficient information on the length of time they were unable to perform activities of daily living. According to some medical providers and TSGLI staff we interviewed, notes in a servicemember's medical file may not indicate whether the servicemember was able to perform activities of daily living because such notes are often oriented toward treatment and recovery, rather than documenting the inability to perform certain activities. Medical providers said that occupational therapists may perform assessments of activities of daily living for servicemembers, but that these may only indicate a servicemember's functional ability at one point in time, rather than at the specified intervals of 15, 30, 60, or 90 days as required by TSGLI. Furthermore, occupational therapy may not occur until after a servicemember's injuries have been stabilized, which may be after the qualifying period for documenting the inability to perform the activities of daily living as required by TSGLI. In addition, VA and TSGLI officials told us that challenges in documenting loss of activities of daily living may have been greater for servicemembers whose injuries occurred prior to the implementation of the program because medical providers at major medical facilities may not have routinely documented the loss of activities of daily living. Finally, medical documentation may not have clearly stated that the servicemember's inability to perform activities of daily living was directly related to his or her traumatic brain injury, although such a link is necessary to establish a servicemember's eligibility for TSGLI.

VA has recognized that documenting the loss of activities of daily living for traumatic brain injury is difficult, and made a change in the program to create another way for servicemembers to qualify for the minimum TSGLI benefit. In its year-one review of the program, VA stated that a 15-day continuous hospital stay from the time of the traumatic brain injury is equivalent to the first 15 days of the inability to perform activities of daily living. As a result, servicemembers with traumatic brain injury who can document a 15-day hospital stay are now eligible for a TSGLI benefit of $25,000. This change in eligibility criteria, effective in November 2008, expands access to the TSGLI program for servicemembers with traumatic brain injury.[22] For example, one of the servicemembers we interviewed had a traumatic brain injury in addition to facial fractures and lacerations due to a blast from an improvised explosive device in Iraq. He was denied for TSGLI because he was able to document the loss of only one activity of daily living— eating—but may qualify under the revised criteria because he told us he was an inpatient for a month at a major medical treatment facility.

DOD and VA officials told us that the services are reviewing all claims that were denied or approved for less than the maximum amount to determine if the servicemembers are now eligible for an initial or higher TSGLI payment under the clarified guidance for the activities of daily living criteria and the revised eligibility criteria. Officials also told us they were exploring options, such as data matches with military and VA injury tracking systems, to identify servicemembers who never applied for TSGLI but may now be eligible.[23]

Conclusions

Three years after the creation of the TSGLI program, DOD and VA have taken a number of important, proactive steps to improve the program for all servicemembers, including those with traumatic brain injury. DOD and VA efforts to improve program outreach, revise eligibility criteria, and clarify guidance for assessing the inability to perform activities of daily living will help expand access to the program to more servicemembers with traumatic brain injury. However, given the large population of servicemembers with traumatic brain injury, determining who is eligible for TSGLI on the basis of the activities of daily living may continue to present challenges because such assessments involve subjectivity and require adequate, timely documentation of a servicemember's functional abilities. Furthermore, there is no alternative, objective test to quantify loss of functioning due to traumatic brain injury. The military medical community is still learning about traumatic brain injury and a great deal of research is ongoing that might ultimately bring new tools for measuring traumatic brain injury and understanding its short- and long-term effects on individuals' lives. This research could prove useful to VA as the agency seeks to continuously improve the TSGLI program for servicemembers with traumatic brain injury.

Without a systematic quality assurance review process, DOD and VA lack information on whether the services are consistently applying the program eligibility criteria and making accurate decisions on servicemembers' claims. Furthermore, the agencies lack assurance that servicemembers with similar injuries, but in different services, are receiving equitable treatment with respect to the TSGLI program.

In addition, by not addressing a software limitation that excludes some traumatic brain injury denials from its data, VA lacks complete information on the total universe of traumatic brain injury claimants and the disposition of their claims. Such information is important for understanding how well the program is working and for making any adjustments to further enhance program performance. Finally, given that the intent of the program is to provide a quick benefit to address servicemembers' needs while they recover from their traumatic injuries, timely decisions are important. While the services have goals for reviewing and making decisions on servicemembers' claims and report they are exceeding these goals, DOD and VA are unable to determine whether they are actually meeting these goals without reliable data. Furthermore, absent timeliness data broken out by type of injury, DOD and VA are unable to determine whether servicemembers with traumatic brain injury are experiencing unnecessary delays. Moreover, without better data, VA and the services lack a reliable baseline from which to determine whether new initiatives to improve the TSGLI program have the desired effect.

Recommendations for Executive Action

To improve management of the Servicemembers' Group Life Insurance Traumatic Injury Protection Program (known as TSGLI) and ensure that all injured servicemembers receive accurate, consistent, and timely treatment, we recommend that the Secretary of Veterans Affairs work with the Secretary of Defense and the branches of service to take the following two actions:

- Implement a systematic quality assurance review process to help ensure that TSGLI benefit decisions are accurate and consistent within and across the services. For example, VA could expand its planned review of a sample of TSGLI claim decisions into a systematic, ongoing quality assurance review process.
- Take steps to ensure that the data required to assess approval rates for traumatic brain injury and the timeliness of key steps in the TSGLI claims process are reliable and comprehensive.

Appendix I. Objectives, Scope, and Methodology

The objectives of our report were to examine (1) the approval rate of Servicemembers' Group Life Insurance Traumatic Injury Protection Program (TSGLI) claims for traumatic brain injury, and whether the Department of Defense (DOD) and the Department of Veterans Affairs (VA) have assurance that claims are processed accurately, consistently, and in a timely manner and (2) any challenges servicemembers with traumatic brain injury may have faced in accessing TSGLI benefits, and the extent to which DOD and VA have taken steps to address such challenges.

Data Reliability and Quality Assurance

To address the first objective, we analyzed data VA gathered from its contractor, the Office of Servicemembers' Group Life Insurance (OSGLI), and the services on the number of claimants and the final disposition and timeliness of their claims since the program's inception. We restricted our scope to the Air Force, Army, Marine Corps, and Navy because these four services represent nearly all (99.9 percent) of the TSGLI applications filed.[24]

To assess the reliability of data from OSGLI, the primary entity responsible for recording data for the TSGLI program, we interviewed officials from VA and OSGLI at the latter's offices in Roseland, New Jersey. OSGLI officials demonstrated their data entry procedures and explained their quality review processes. In addition, we randomly selected and reviewed 100 TSGLI claimants' paper claim files, representing 1 percent of all TSGLI claimants whose claims were decided through June 30, 2008. We compared the data on the claim forms with the data in OSGLI's electronic database. On the basis of this review, we found that the data were sufficiently reliable to report the number of claimants and the final disposition of their claims. However, we found a number of limitations with respect to the number of traumatic brain injury claimants and their dispositions. For example, (1) OSGLI and VA do not include all traumatic brain injury denials in the traumatic brain injury category in their data, which makes the actual approval rate lower than reported and (2) the data system can only record one claim and one primary injury per claimant.

To assess the reliability of data from the monthly reports the services provide to VA, we interviewed TSGLI officials at the Air Force, Army, Marine Corps, and Navy about the procedures they have in place to ensure that the electronic data they keep are accurate. We found that, while the services perform some spot checks of these data before sending them to VA, they do not match the electronic data reported to paper claim files. Also, the internal control procedures were not robust enough to prevent a number of errors in the data. When VA provided us with the data from the services as of June 30, 2008, VA noted that they found that the electronic records for 277 out of 707 claims contained missing or out of sequence dates for key steps along the process. For example, 43 records had key dates missing, such as the date the servicemember signed his or her claim. In addition, for 95 records, the date recorded for the servicemember's signature on the claim form was prior to the recorded date of the servicemember's injury. Furthermore, VA shared that there had been some confusion among the services over the definition of a key data element, the date of loss.[25] For some cases we reviewed, the dates in this field did not match dates for the same field in VA's central data system, even though data for both datasets came from the same source—submitted claim applications.

We interviewed VA officials to assess the reliability of a one-time study on the timeliness of key steps in the claims process. VA collected the data from this study from a random sample of 238 claim forms, stratified by injury. According to VA officials, this study represented claims decided between December 1, 2005, and December 31, 2006, for injuries that occurred after the effective date of the program on December 1, 2005, known as prospective claims. We found these data to be reliable and representative of claimants with traumatic brain injury for that period.

Finally, we interviewed DOD, VA, service branch, and OSGLI officials on the procedures in place to ensure accuracy and consistency of decision making. Additionally, we reviewed TSGLI procedure guides.

Challenges for Servicemembers with Traumatic Brain Injury

To address the second objective, we interviewed DOD and VA officials and reviewed TSGLI enacting legislation and regulations, program guidance issued by DOD, VA, and the services as well as the program procedural guide, published August 2007. We also reviewed VA's year-one review of the TSGLI program, published in July 2008, and related materials, including interim final regulations, VA's revised procedural guide, and the new TSGLI claim form. In addition, we attended a September 2008 training session for TSGLI officials and other relevant staff on the proposed changes in guidance and changes to eligibility criteria.

We interviewed TSGLI officials responsible for adjudicating and certifying claims and conducting outreach to prospective claimants at the Army, Air Force, Marine Corps, and Navy to learn about how they decide claims; understand the policies each service has in place to guide the disposition of claims; and determine what, if any, challenges complicate the adjudication process, specifically for servicemembers with traumatic brain injury.

We discussed challenges in accessing TSGLI benefits with 31 servicemembers with traumatic brain injury or their family members, in both group and individual interviews. These servicemembers represented those who (1) had not yet applied for TSGLI benefits, (2) were in the process of applying for TSGLI benefits, (3) had applied and been approved for TSGLI benefits, or (4) had applied and been denied for TSGLI benefits. The servicemembers we interviewed included both retroactive claimants and prospective claimants. Specifically, we discussed these challenges with servicemembers with traumatic brain injury and, in some cases, their family members; medical providers; and service branch TSGLI staff at the following four medical treatment facilities: Brooke Army Medical Center at Fort Sam Houston in Texas; National Naval Medical Center, Bethesda, Maryland; Walter Reed Army Medical Center, Washington, D.C.; and the Polytrauma Rehabilitation Center at the Hunter Holmes McGuire VA Medical Center, Richmond, Virginia. We selected these sites because they represent three of DOD's larger medical treatment facilities for traumatic brain injury cases and one of VA's four designated traumatic brain injury centers. We conducted 4 group interviews with 14 servicemembers at Brooke Army Medical Center and 1 group interview with 6 servicemembers at Walter Reed Army Medical Center. We conducted six individual interviews with servicemembers or family members at the other two treatment facilities. We also completed five telephone interviews with servicemembers or their family members. To conduct these interviews, we drew a random sample of 60 servicemembers from the population of the 821 servicemembers who applied for TSGLI as of June 30, 2008, under the traumatic brain injury category, stratified to include (1) denied and approved claimants, (2) retroactive and prospective claimants, and (3) claimants from each of the services. From that random sample, we contacted servicemembers on the list until we completed five interviews. Servicemembers were removed from the list if their telephones had been disconnected or were no longer valid, they were not living in the United States, or they could not be reached after two separate attempts to contact them.

In addition, we discussed the nature of traumatic brain injury and challenges that servicemembers with traumatic brain injury may face in applying for TSGLI with medical professionals at the Defense and Veterans Brain Injury Center as well as the Brain Injury Association of America. We also interviewed representatives from three military and veterans' advocacy groups—Iraq and Afghanistan Veterans of America, Disabled American Veterans, and the Wounded Warrior Project.

Furthermore, we reviewed data from a customer satisfaction survey of servicemembers who applied for TSGLI benefits conducted by VA's contractor and found these data to be reliable for our purposes. We confirmed that the sample population was representative of the TSGLI population and verified that the contact method for the interview and questions asked did not bias the results.

Appendix II. Comments from the Department of Defense

UNDER SECRETARY OF DEFENSE
4000 DEFENSE PENTAGON
WASHINGTON, D.C. 20301-4000

DEC 2 3

PERSONNEL AND
READINESS

Mr. Daniel Bertoni
Director, Education, Workforce,
and Income Security Issues
U.S. Government Accountability Office
441 G Street, NW
Washington, D.C. 20548

Dear Mr. Bertoni:

This is the Department of Defense (DoD) response to the GAO draft report, "TRAUMATIC BRAIN INJURY: Better DoD and VA Oversight Can Help Ensure More Accurate, Consistent, and Timely Decisions for Traumatic Injury Insurance Program," dated November 20, 2008, (GAO Code 130823/GAO-09-108).

The Department notes GAO has retitled the draft report by its primary finding, which does not address the initial study purpose - Traumatic Group Life Insurance Program for Service members with Traumatic Brain Injury. Our preference is that the title be amended to reflect the report content, not a single finding.

Examination of the approval rates for Traumatic Servicemembers' Group Life Insurance (TSGLI) claims submitted for Traumatic Brain Injury may not provide an accurate assessment of the program. Many members, especially early in the TSGLI program, were encouraged to submit claims even if they believed that the claim would ultimately be denied. The opinion that, "I'll make them tell me 'no'" was encouraged by the Services early in the program to ensure that members did not slip through the eligibility process. However, it resulted in claim denial rates that were inflated.

The report states that the Department of Veterans Affairs (VA) attributes the higher approval rate experienced by the Marine Corps as likely due to efforts to place TSGLI staff in medical facilities. However, the report notes that without a quality assurance review, there is no way to accurately determine the reason for the difference. We believe that a comparison of the claim approval rates before placement of TSGLI staff in medical facilities to the rates experienced after placement of staff would indicate a significant improvement. Indeed, that comparison, between pre-placement and post-placement of TSGLI personnel in medical facilities, led the DoD to encourage other military departments to make the same personnel transfers. The random sample of 100 cases likely included claim experiences that occurred both before and after the process was improved.

We agree that a quality assurance review process would help to ensure that claim examination is accurate and consistent. Although the VA and DoD have communicated regularly on TSGLI issues through monthly conference calls and routine correspondence, a formal review process does not exist. Further, the VA is the logical agency to staff and fund the reviewing body since they are the agency tasked in Title 38 to promulgate regulations in support of TSGLI.

Please address comments or questions to Mr. Tim Fowlkes at (703) 697-3793, or tim.fowlkes@osd.mil.

Sincerely,

David S. C. Chu

Enclosure:
Formal Comments

GAO DRAFT REPORT – Dated November 20, 2008
GAO CODE 130823/GAO-09-108

"TRAUMATIC BRAIN INJURY: Better DoD and VA Oversight Can Help Ensure More Accurate, Consistent, and Timely Decisions for Traumatic Injury Insurance Program"

DEPARTMENT OF DEFENSE COMMENTS
TO THE RECOMMENDATIONS

RECOMMENDATION 1: The GAO recommends that the Secretary of Veterans Affairs work with the Secretary of Defense and the branches of Service to implement a systematic quality assurance review process to help ensure that the Servicemembers' Group Life Insurance Traumatic Injury Protection Program (TSGLI) benefit decisions are accurate and consistent within and across the branches of Service.

DOD RESPONSE: Concur. An increased level of quality assurance will benefit the TSGLI program. Because some of the TSGLI implementing regulations and procedural guidance leave room for interpretation, especially those sections related to Traumatic Brain Injury (TBI) and Post Traumatic Stress Disorder (PTSD), a quality assurance review process should improve the overall program. In addition, the revision to TSGLI policy, published as a result of the Year One Review on November 26, 2008 should greatly improve consistency among the Services.

RECOMMENDATION 2: The GAO recommended that the Secretary of Veterans Affairs work with the Secretary of Defense and the branches of Service to take steps to ensure the data required to assess approval rates for traumatic brain injury and the timeliness of key steps in the Servicemembers' Group Life Insurance Traumatic Injury Protection Program (TSGLI) claims process are reliable and comprehensive.

DOD RESPONSE: Concur. The report accurately references the laudable efforts that DOD has taken to assist Soldiers in initiating claims, as well as establishing and documenting their eligibility. Significant progress has been made through DoD and VA efforts to document and report the timeliness of TSGLI claim submission and the payment of claims, however, room for

Appendix III. Comments from the Department of Veterans Affairs

THE SECRETARY OF VETERANS AFFAIRS
WASHINGTON

December 22, 2008

Mr. Daniel Bertoni
Director
Education, Workforce and
  Income Security Issues
U.S. Government Accountability Office
441 G Street, NW
Washington, DC 20548

Dear Mr. Bertoni:

The Department of Veterans Affairs (VA) has reviewed the Government Accountability Office's (GAO) draft report, *TRAUMATIC BRAIN INJURY: Better DOD and VA Oversight Can Help Ensure More Accurate, Consistent, and Timely Decisions for Traumatic Injury Insurance Program* (GAO-09-108) and generally agrees with its findings and recommendations.

VA and Department of Defense leadership remain committed to the Traumatic Injury Insurance Program and to making necessary improvements to the program to address the short-term financial burdens traumatically injured service members and their families face. The enclosure discusses GAO's recommendations in detail. It also suggests some technical clarification for the report's overall accuracy. VA appreciates the opportunity to comment on your draft report.

Sincerely yours,

James B. Peake, M.D.

Enclosure

Department of Veterans Affairs (VA)
Response to GAO Draft Report
TRAUMATIC BRAIN INJURY: Better DOD and VA Oversight Can Help Ensure More Accurate, Consistent, and Timely Decisions for Traumatic Injury Insurance Program
(GAO-09-108)

GAO Recommendations:

To improve management of the Servicemembers' Group Life Insurance Traumatic Injury Protection Program (known as TSGLI) and ensure that all injured service members receive consistent, accurate, and timely treatment, GAO recommends that the Secretary of Veterans Affairs work with the Secretary of Defense and the branches of service to take the following two actions:

Recommendation 1: Implement a systematic quality assurance review process to help ensure that TSGLI benefit decisions are accurate and consistent within and across the branches of service. For example, VBA could expand its planned reviews of a sample of TSGLI claim decisions into a systematic, ongoing quality assurance review.

Response: Concur. However, we believe that the underlying finding that, "...DOD and VBA lack assurance that TSGLI decisions are accurate and consistent across the services...," while true as stated, is misleading without clarification. While it is accurate to say there has been no statistically valid sampling to determine consistency among branches of service, there have been a number of measures in place since the beginning of the program to promote accuracy and consistency.

When the Office of Servicemembers' Group Life Insurance (OSGLI) began paying TSGLI claims in December 2005, claims examiners reviewed medical records and other documentation to ensure that the claim had been adjudicated properly by the branch of service. In addition, 100 percent of TSGLI claims were subject to OSGLI's Internal Quality Review process for accuracy in the preparation of the award. By the summer of 2006, the potential error rate for TSGLI claims was reduced significantly from December 2005, when the program began, and the claims examiners, although continuing to closely review the claims, no longer received or reviewed any attending medical documentation. Furthermore, the percentage of TSGLI claims reviewed was reduced to 25 percent—the same percentage of Servicemembers' Group Life Insurance death claims that go through OSGLI's Quality Review. This review however, does not check for consistency of decisions across the branches of service.

Additionally, the Veterans Benefits Administration (VBA) produced and distributed to each branch of service a TSGLI Procedures Guide, which provided detailed procedures and guidance on all aspects of the program, and, VBA provided training to the branches regarding the guide.

Department of Veterans Affairs (VA)
Response to GAO Draft Report
TRAUMATIC BRAIN INJURY: Better DOD and VA Oversight Can Help Ensure
More Accurate, Consistent, and Timely Decisions for Traumatic Injury
Insurance Program
(GAO-09-108)
(Continued)

Finally, VBA and OSGLI held weekly (then bi-weekly and ultimately monthly) conference calls with all of the branches of service participating at the same time. The purpose of these calls was to discuss issues related to the program and how they were addressed in the Procedures Guide, and to discuss policy and concepts involving novel issues or unusual claims. These issues were raised and guidance was provided to ensure that all branches were handling case decisions consistently.

During the course of the Year-One Review, VBA recognized the need for a validation of the accuracy and consistency of case decisions made by the branches of service and began discussions about developing and implementing a statistically valid post-adjudicative review process. Accordingly, VBA is in the process of developing an integrated quality assurance review process that will include the branches of service, OSGLI and VBA. This review will include both in-process controls to look at the accuracy and consistency of all cases before they are paid or a denial letter is sent, and a post-adjudicative, statistically valid review of a sample of cases to validate the in-process review. The review process will also include a detailed feedback mechanism for the branches of service to ensure they make procedural adjustments as necessary. VBA anticipates full implementation of this recommendation by July 1, 2009.

Recommendation 2: Take steps to ensure the data required to assess approval rates for traumatic brain injury and the timeliness of key steps in the TSGLI claims process are reliable and comprehensive.

Response: Concur. In its report, GAO states that the TSGLI approval rate for traumatic brain injury (TBI) claims may be lower than documented because VBA's data does not include all denials for TBI. As GAO indicates, this is due to a current system limitation that does not allow claims to be recorded in the TBI category unless the medical provider indicates a loss of at least one of the six activities of daily living. System enhancements are being implemented that will allow such claims to be captured as TBI claims.

GAO's report states that DOD and VBA lack reliable, sufficient data to oversee the timeliness of the TSGLI claims process. Although VBA believes the reported timeliness of TSGLI claims from the date of injury to the date of payment is generally accurate, during the course of the Year-One Review, VBA identified problems with the TSGLI timeliness reports and began working with the branches of service to reconcile the timeliness data

---

Department of Veterans Affairs (VA)
Response to GAO Draft Report
**TRAUMATIC BRAIN INJURY: Better DOD and VA Oversight Can Help Ensure
More Accurate, Consistent, and Timely Decisions for Traumatic Injury
Insurance Program**
(GAO-09-108)
(Continued)

they were providing. VBA is implementing a systematic reconciliation process by which reports with missing or inaccurate numbers are returned to the branches of service for correction. In cases where dates cannot be provided (e.g. service member does not date the form), procedures are being established on how those cases will be handled. VBA is also clarifying definitions of the timeliness milestones within the process (e.g., from date of injury to date claim is submitted, and from date claim is submitted to date the medical professional completes the form, etc.) to ensure that all branches of service understand and report dates accurately and consistently. Accurate interim milestones will help VBA and the branches make further improvements in the overall timeliness of processing TSGLI claims.

GAO states in its report that the data VBA collects from the branches of service do not break out claims by injury type, and as a result, DOD and VBA lack information on how long it takes the branches of service to make decisions on TBI claims (and by inference other categories of losses). In response, VBA is modifying the process to incorporate injury type into the timeliness data so timeliness can be calculated by injury type. VBA anticipates full implementation of this recommendation by September 30, 2009.

End Notes

[1] This RAND estimate is based on a survey of a representative sample drawn from the population of all those who have been deployed for Operation Enduring Freedom and Operation Iraqi Freedom. Of the 1,965 respondents, 19.5 percent reported experiencing a probable traumatic brain injury during deployment.

[2] Our review focused on the Air Force, Army, Marine Corps, and Navy because these services represent almost all of the TSGLI claims filed as of June 30, 2008. However, we have included data from Coast Guard claims in our analyses.

[3] According to the Defense and Veterans Brain Injury Center, less is known about the nature of combat-related traumatic brain injury and the short- and long-term outcomes for servicemembers, particularly those who suffered brain injuries caused by blasts.

[4] Pub. L. No. 109-13 (2005); 38 U.S.C. § 1980A.

[5] All servicemembers paying premiums into the Servicemembers' Group Life Insurance Program are automatically covered by TSGLI while they are in service. According to the VA's *Performance and Accountability Report* for fiscal year 2008, 99 percent of servicemembers were enrolled in the Servicemembers' Group Life Insurance Program.

[6] Servicemembers may be eligible for retroactive benefits if their injuries occurred during this time period while they were deployed outside of the United States on orders in support of

·   Operation Enduring Freedom or Operation Iraqi Freedom or while they were serving in a geographic location that qualified them for the Combat Zone Tax Exclusion.

[7] For the purposes of this chapter, we will primarily use the term injury. However, it is important to note that TSGLI provides compensation for the eligible losses that result from these injuries—such as a loss of hand or foot or, in the case of traumatic brain injury, the loss of the ability to perform activities of daily living—rather than for the injuries themselves.

[8] VA officials explained this criterion by noting that TSGLI was not intended to serve as a death benefit, and that requiring claimants to survive at least 7 days preserves this intent.

[9] Injuries caused by a mental disorder, a mental or physical illness or disease—unless caused by a pyogenic (pus forming, often from a wound) infection, biological, chemical, or radiological weapon—or attempted suicide are not covered by TSGLI. Furthermore, injuries sustained while committing or attempting to commit a felony and injuries caused by self-inflicted wounds; medical or surgical treatment of an illness or disease; or willful use of an illegal or controlled substance, unless administered or consumed on the advice of a medical professional, are not covered.

[10] For example, a servicemember may have traumatic brain injury causing an inability to perform activities of daily living for 30 days, in addition to an amputation of one foot. If found eligible for TSGLI, he or she would receive $50,000 for traumatic brain injury and $50,000 for the loss of one foot, for a total of $100,000. However, according to TSGLI procedures, a servicemember may not combine payment for an injury under the other traumatic injury category with payment for an injury in another category.

[11] VA initially began making payments under an interim final rule published in the *Federal Register* on December 22, 2005. The final rules were published on March 8, 2007 (38 C.F.R. Part 9).

[12] According to agency officials, the purpose of these conference calls is to discuss policy issues and unusual cases.

[13] There are other denials for traumatic brain injury that also are not reflected in VA's central data system because this system only records one claim per claimant and one primary injury category. For example, a previously denied claim for traumatic brain injury may not appear in VA's data if a later claim for a different injury was approved for that individual. As a result, data may not reflect all servicemembers who claimed a traumatic brain injury. However, officials told us that tracking the number of servicemembers who receive benefits is a better measure of the program's impact than tracking individual claims.

[14] The data do not reflect denials that are in the process of being appealed.

[15] In our limited review of a small sample of claim forms, traumatic brain injury claims were denied due to a lack of medical documentation to support the loss of ability to perform activities of daily living or because the servicemembers' injuries occurred in a non-combat zone prior to the effective date of the program, December 1, 2005.

[16] According to the *Standards for Internal Control in the Federal Government*, internal control monitoring—one of five internal control activities—should assess the quality of performance over time. Internal controls should generally be designed to ensure that ongoing monitoring occurs in the course of normal operations, including regular management and supervisory activities, comparisons, reconciliations, and other actions people take in performing their duties. See GAO, *Standards for Internal Control in the Federal Government*, GAO/AIMD-00-21.3.1 (Washington, D.C.: November 1999).

[17] VA officials noted that early in the TSGLI program, claims examiners from the Office of Servicemembers' Group Life Insurance reviewed medical documentation to ensure the claim had been adjudicated properly by the services. However, as of the summer of 2006, claims examiners no longer receive or review medical documentation.

[18] In commenting on our draft report, DOD noted that it believed a comparison of the approval rates before and after placing TSGLI staff in medical treatment facilities would show a significant improvement. However, neither DOD nor VA has conducted such an evaluation

that would control for other factors that could have contributed to different approval rates between the two services.

[19] Government internal control standards require agencies to have internal control activities to help ensure that data on the entire process or life cycle of a transaction are complete and accurate to support decision making. See GAO/AIMD-00-21.3.1.

[20] In its Year-One Review of the TSGLI program, VA found that some servicemembers may have delayed applying for TSGLI because it would have prevented them from continuing to receive Combat-related Injury and Rehabilitation Pay. However, Combat-related Injury and Rehabilitation Pay has been replaced by the Pay and Allowances Continuation Program, which is not linked to the receipt of a TSGLI benefit.

[21] According to VA's revised TSGLI procedural guide, stand-by assistance is defined as when a patient requires someone to be within arm's reach because the patient's ability fluctuates and physical or verbal assistance may be needed.

[22] This will also expand access to the program for servicemembers with a 15-day hospital stay for other traumatic injuries. The 15-day hospital stay will substitute for the first eligibility period for the other traumatic injury category, which is 30 days.

[23] VA officials told us they are conducting data mining with the Joint Patient Tracking and Veterans Tracking Applications to identify veterans who may now be eligible for TSGLI.

[24] However, when reporting TSGLI data, we included the eight claims that have been filed in the Coast Guard.

[25] The date of loss is the date a servicemember becomes eligible for the TSGLI program. For example, a servicemember with traumatic brain injury may be eligible for TSGLI benefits after he or she is unable to perform the activities of daily living for at least 15 days.

In: Hidden Wounds: Traumatic Brain...   ISBN: 978-1-61122-415-3
Editor: Joseph R. Phillips   © 2011 Nova Science Publishers, Inc.

Chapter 4

PolyTrauma-Traumatic Brain Injury (TBI) System of Care

Department of Veterans Affairs

1. **REASON FOR ISSUE:** This Veterans Health Administration (VHA) Directive defines the policy for the Polytrauma-Traumatic Brain Injury (TBI) System of Care.
2. **BACKGROUND**
   a. Blast injuries resulting in polytrauma and TBI are among the most frequent combat-related injuries from Operation Enduring Freedom (OEF) and Operation Iraqi Freedom (OIF). Polytrauma and TBI can also occur as a result of non-combat events, such as motor vehicle accidents. To ensure that the needs of injured servicemembers and Veterans are met, VHA developed a Polytrauma-TBI System of Care that provides specialized rehabilitation care for Veterans and servicemembers with polytrauma and TBI. The system is designed to balance the need for highly-specialized expertise with the need for accessibility.
   b. **Definitions**
      (1) **Polytrauma.** Polytrauma is defined as two or more injuries sustained in the same incident that affect multiple body parts or organ systems and result in physical, cognitive, psychological, or psychosocial impairments and functional

disabilities. TBI frequently occurs as part of the polytrauma spectrum in combination with other disabling conditions, such as amputations, burns, pain, fractures, auditory and visual impairments, post traumatic stress disorder (PTSD), and other mental health conditions. When present, injury to the brain is often the impairment that dictates the course of rehabilitation due to the nature of the cognitive, emotional, and behavioral deficits related to TBI.

(2) **TBI.** TBI is defined as traumatically induced structural injury or physiological disruption of brain function as a result of an external force. Injuries can be penetrating or closed, and the latter can be mild, moderate, or severe. Severity level of the TBI is determined by using the following measurements at the time of the injury: Glasgow Coma Scale (GCS) score, length of loss of consciousness (LOC), and length of post-traumatic amnesia (PTA).

c. The spectrum of TBI injuries is highly variable. The majority of TBIs due to blast or other mechanisms are mild, and most patients recover within days or weeks. When rapidly and appropriately managed, mild TBI, often called concussion, tends to resolve with no or only minimal functional sequelae. A small percentage of persons with mild TBI have symptoms that require specialized rehabilitation services to manage acute problems and to prevent long-term sequelae. On the other hand, persons with moderate to severe TBI generally require intensive inpatient rehabilitation. Many of these individuals may have some permanent functional sequelae that can be significantly reduced with timely and appropriate services. Persons with severe TBI will often have functionally devastating injuries that may cause impairments that require life long assistance with activities of daily living. Again, early and specialized care can reduce acute and long-term medical and functional impairments.

d. In 2004, Congress passed Public Law 108-422, The Veterans Health Programs Improvement Act of 2004, Section 302, which directed the Department of Veterans Affairs (VA) to designate an appropriate number of cooperative centers for clinical care, consultation, research and education activities on complex TBI and Polytrauma associated with combat injuries. Further, the Conference Report for Public Law 108-447 (Conference Report on H.R. 4818, Report 108-792) directs VA to implement a new initiative to ensure that returning war Veterans with loss of limb and other severe and lasting injuries have access to the best of both modern medicine and integrative holistic therapies. In 2008, to further meet the needs of servicemembers and Veterans in combat operations, Title 38 United States Code sections 1710D, 1710D, and 1710E were enacted.

e. In response VA developed the Polytrauma- TBI System of Care (PSC), that integrates specialized rehabilitation services available at regional centers, Veterans Integrated Service (VISN) sites, and at local VA medical centers. Polytrauma and TBI rehabilitation care is provided at the facility closest to the Veteran's home that has the expertise necessary to manage the Veteran's rehabilitation, physical, and mental health needs. The tiered PSC includes four components or levels of care:

(1) **Polytrauma Rehabilitation Centers (PRC).** PRCs are located at the VA medical centers in Minneapolis, MN; Palo Alto, CA; Richmond, VA; and Tampa, FL. *NOTE: A fifth PRC has been designated at the San Antonio, TX VA Medical Center and is in the design phase.* The PRCs serve as regional referral centers for acute medical and rehabilitation care, and as hubs for research and education related to Polytrauma and TBI. They provide a continuum of rehabilitation services that include: specialized "emerging consciousness" programs, comprehensive acute rehabilitation care for complex and severe polytraumatic injuries, outpatient programs, and residential transitional rehabilitation programs (PTRP).

(a) PRCs have a minimum of twelve dedicated comprehensive rehabilitation beds located contiguously on a specialized unit designed for rehabilitation, with a dedicated staff of highly-trained rehabilitation specialists (see Att. A). Four of the beds on the inpatient PRC units are used for the Emerging Consciousness Program that was developed for minimally-responsive patients. In addition, the PRCs have a minimum of ten dedicated Transitional Rehabilitation beds located in a specially-designed unit within, or in close proximity to, the medical center, i.e., on the medical center campus (see Att. B).

(b) PRCs maintain accreditation by the Commission on Accreditation of Rehabilitation Facilities (CARF) for comprehensive inpatient medical rehabilitation, brain injury rehabilitation, and residential rehabilitation. The needed Prosthetic and Orthotic Laboratories are accredited by the American Board for Certification in Orthotics and Prosthetics, Inc. (ABC), or the Board for Orthotist or Prosthetist Certification (BOC).

(c) Dedicated consultative services in medical and surgical specialties are available to provide care for patients with a high degree of medical complexity and acuity (see Att. C).

(d) Nursing and social work care managers coordinate clinical and support services for patients and their families.

(e) PRCs are responsible for:

1. Providing a comfortable age appropriate envir-nment of care, and maintaining state-of-the-art equipment and technology for advanced rehab-ilitation practice.

2. Playing a leadership role in the development of best practice models for polytrauma and TBI and rehabilitation.

3. Collaborating in research that addresses the sequelae of polytrauma and TBI, and the means of improving the diagnosis, treatment, and prevention of such sequelae.

4. Collaboratively developing and conducting national level educational programs for providers, as well as patients and families in the areas of polytrauma and TBI.

5. Maintaining affiliations with local academic medical programs in the areas of medical rehabilitation and allied health.

(2) **Polytrauma Network Sites (PNS).** PNSs provide key components of post-acute rehabilitation care for individuals with polytrauma and TBI including, but not limited to

inpatient and outpatient rehabilitation, and day programs. PNSs are located in each of VA's 21 VISNs (see Att. F).

(a) PNSs have an interdisciplinary outpatient program that serves Veterans with polytrauma and TBI. A dedicated interdisciplinary team (see Att. D) provides services that include: evaluation, development and management of the rehabilitation and community re-integration plan; interdisciplinary rehabilitation treatment; and coordination of services between VA, the Department of Defense (DOD) and other governmental and private providers.

(b) PNSs maintain CARF accreditation of their inpatient bed unit for comprehensive inpatient medical rehabilitation. When polytrauma and TBI patients are admitted for inpatient care, the PNS team will have the lead in the development and management of the plan of care.

(c) Prosthetic and Orthotic Laboratories are accredited by the ABC or the BOC.

(d) PNS interdisciplinary teams conduct comprehensive evaluations of patients with positive TBI screens, and develop rehabilitation and community re-integration plans as indicated.

(e) Nursing and social work care managers coordinate clinical and support services for patients and their families.

(f) PNSs provide a comfortable age appropriate environment of care, and maintain state-of-the-art equipment and technology for advanced rehabilitation practice.

(g) PNSs serve as coordinating centers for polytrauma and TBI care within their respective VISN. This includes tracking high risk patients, standardization of care via site visits and teleconferences, and acting as a referral source for complex patients from across the VISN.

(h) PNSs collaboratively develop and conduct VISN-level educational programs for providers as well as patients and families in the areas of polytrauma and TBI.

(i) PNSs collaborate in tracking VISN-level outcome data and performance monitors for polytrauma and TBI.

(3) **Polytrauma Support Clinic Team (PSCT).** PSCTs provide interdisciplinary outpatient rehabilitation services for Veterans and active duty servicemembers with mild and or stable functional deficits from TBI and polytrauma (see Att. F).

    (a) A dedicated interdisciplinary outpatient team (see Att. E) provides specialty rehabilitation care including evaluation, development of a treatment plan, inter-disciplinary rehabilitation treatment, and long-term management of patients with ongoing rehabilitation needs.

    (b) Nursing and social work case managers coordinate clinical and support services for patients and their families.

    (c) PSCTs conduct comprehensive evaluations of patients with positive TBI screens, and develop rehabilitation and community re-integration plans, as indicated.

(4) **Polytrauma Points of Contact (PPOC).** A PPOC is identified in every VA facility that is not otherwise designated as one of the PSC components described. The PPOC ensures that patients with polytrauma and TBI are referred to a facility or program capable of providing the level of rehabilitation services required. PPOCs commonly refer to the PNS and PSCTs within their VISN (see Att. F).

f.   **Rehabilitation Care in the PSC.** The PSC is dedicated to providing rehabilitation services that restore physical, intellectual, communicative, psychosocial and vocational skills, and to facilitating the transfer of those skills from the hospital setting to daily life. Such services include, but are not limited to, inpatient rehabilitation, outpatient rehabilitation, emerging consciousness programs, transitional rehabilitation, day programs, and community re-entry programs. The PSC also manages ongoing and emerging rehabilitation and psychosocial needs of Veterans with polytrauma and TBI. This includes ongoing follow up and treatment, case management, coordination of services, monitoring implementation of the treatment plan, overseeing the quality and intensity of VA and non-VA services, and providing education and support for patients and caregivers.

3. **POLICY:** It is VHA's policy that the PSC provide and manage the full-range of rehabilitation care for all eligible Veterans and active duty servicemembers who sustained polytrauma and TBI.

4. **ACTION**

   a. **Under Secretary for Health.** The Under Secretary for Health is responsible for approving any proposed changes to the PSC including, but not limited to, changes in mission, staffing, bed level, reduction of clinical services, reorganization, and changes in clinical staff.

   b. **Principal Under Secretary for Health.** The Principal Under Secretary for Health is responsible for providing guidance and ensuring compliance for any program office changes, to include changes in mission, staffing, bed levels, and clinical services.

   c. **Physical Medicine and Rehabilitation Services (PM&RS) National Program Director.** The PM&RS National Program Director is responsible for:

   (1) Providing national program leadership for the PSC;

   (2) Identifying the scope of rehabilitation services provided by the PSC;

   (3) Establishing an effective service delivery model;

   (4) Providing referral and clinical care guidance;

   (5) Representing VHA on matters concerning polytrauma and TBI rehabilitation;

   (6) Monitoring the PSC with regard to capacity, clinical care outcomes, and costs;

   (7) Providing involvement with VISN leadership in designating the facilities participating in the PSC;

   (8) Reviewing and recommending approval of new programs; and

   (9) Reviewing proposed program changes with the Chief Officer for Patient Care Services, Principal Deputy Under Secretary for Health, Deputy Under Secretary for Health for Operations and Management, and other relevant program offices and staff before forwarding recommendations to the Under Secretary for Health.

   d. **VISN Director.** The VISN provides a critical juncture in implementation and support for the PSC, balancing needs for local responsiveness with national consistency and coordination; therefore, the VISN Director, or designee, is responsible for:

(1) Facilitating smooth and efficient access and transfers of care between DOD, VA, and non-VA facilities as Veterans transition to VHA care closer to their home;

(2) Ensuring that appropriate rehabilitation services across the continuum of care, from either VA or non-VA sources, are made available for Veterans with polytrauma and TBI;

(3) Ensuring there is a VISN-wide integrated referral process for polytrauma and TBI care including all medical centers and clinics;

(4) Providing and facilitating necessary communication, resources, and quality improvement efforts to maintain expertise and quality services in the PSC;

(5) Facilitating the education of VHA health care providers regarding the PSC, polytrauma and TBI related health care issues; and

(6) Ensuring proposed changes to PSC programs under their purview are reviewed and approved by the Deputy Under Secretary for Health for Operations and Management, Chief Patient Care Services Officer, Chief Consultant, Rehabilitation Services, National Program Director, PM&RS, and Principal Deputy Under Secretary for Health before forwarding to the Under Secretary for Health for approval.

e. **Facility Director.** Each facility Director, or designee, is responsible for ensuring that:

(1) The VA medical center first contacted for care will facilitate and assist with referral to the nearest appropriate PSC site with the capability of meeting the clinical and rehabilitation care needs;

(2) VA and non-VA inter-facility transfers are timely and follow policy outlined in current VHA policy;

(3) Appropriate specialty care is accessible within a reasonable geographic distance, and making arrangements for non-VA care when such care is not available within VA;

(4) The medical center proactively identifies non-VA community based programs whenever necessary to meet the care needs for Veterans with polytrauma and TBI that cannot be met otherwise. These may include, but are not limited to, outpatient rehabilitation therapies, neurobehavioral

programs, residential transitional rehabilitation, and age appropriate long term care facilities; and

(5) Provisions are made for polytrauma and TBI patients to have basic medical and primary care and emergent medical care. *NOTE: Admission to the local VA facility may take place, but should not be a prerequisite for coordinating arrangements for admission to a PRC or PNS.*

f. **Chief of Staff and Chief Nurse Executive.** The Chief of Staff and Chief Nurse Executive at each VA medical center are responsible for:

(1) Appointing a PM&R physician as Polytrauma-TBI Medical Director at facilities designated as PRC, PNS, or PSCT;

(2) Ensuring that staff is assigned based on the staffing model for each component in the PSC (see Atts. A, B, C, and D);

(3) Monitoring staffing for each component of the PSC and increasing staff to meet local needs and workload demands.

(4) Ensuring that family needs are assessed, and that required resources and support services are made available to meet those needs, as permitted by law and policy;

(5) Ensuring that there is a smooth hand-off of care between facilities and the components of the PSC; and

(6) Developing training initiatives to ensure that staff has the necessary skills to manage this patient population.

g. **Chief, Physical Medicine and Rehabilitation Services.** The Chief, Physical Medicine and Rehabilitation Services, or designee, is responsible for:

(1) Providing clinical care and services to polytrauma and TBI patients consistent with the scope of care of the respective PSC component;

(2) Providing leadership to the interdisciplinary team for patient care and program development;

(3) Assessing family needs and providing support services and education;

(4) Ensuring adequate communication between facilities whenever a transfer of care occurs, including physician-to-physician calls when necessary;

(5) Ensuring that a comprehensive, patient-centered interdisciplinary treatment is developed that sets goals for

recovery and facilitates transitions across settings and programs;

(6) Ensuring that the discharge plan is communicated to all stakeholders involved in patient care and support, e.g., DoD, Care Management and Social Work Service, receiving Military Treatment Facility (MTF), or VHA facility, patient, and family;

(7) Ensuring that written policies and procedures are developed in compliance with all applicable accrediting organizations and VHA program offices, standards and requirements, and that they are reviewed and updated as necessary; and

(8) Managing service-level quality improvement activities that monitor critical aspects of care. An ongoing and continuous evaluation of the program must be conducted to ensure the quality and appropriateness of care provided to patients;

(9) Ensuring that the medical inpatient rehabilitation programs and polytrauma residential rehabilitation programs maintain accreditation by CARF in accordance with VHA Handbook 1170.01. *NOTE: According to the 2008 CARF Medical Rehabilitation Standards Manual: "A program seeking accreditation as a Brain Injury Program must include in the Intent to Survey and the site survey all portions of the program (comprehensive integrated inpatient rehabilitation program, outpatient medical rehabilitation program, home- and community-based rehabilitation program, residential rehabilitation program, and vocational services) that the organization provides and that meet the program description."*

(10) Submitting required data elements to the Rehabilitation Program Office.

h. **Facility OEF-OIF Program Manager.** The facility OEF-OIF Program Manager is responsible for:

(1) Facilitating referrals of Veterans with polytrauma and TBI to the PSC facility that can meet their specialized rehabilitation needs; and

(2) Ensuring that all Veterans with polytrauma and TBI who are treated in one of the PSC components have been assigned a case manager.

5. REFERENCES

a. Public Law 108-422 (Section 302), Centers for Research, Education, and Clinical Activities on Complex Multi-trauma Associated with Combat Injuries.

b. Public Law 108-447, Prosthetics and Integrative Health Care Initiative.

c. Memorandum of Understanding, the Department of Veterans Affairs and the Rehabilitation Accreditation Commission (CARF), February 1, 2002.

d. Title 38 U.S.C. 1710C. Traumatic Brain Injury: Plans for Rehabilitation and Reintegration into the Community.

e. Title 38 U.S.C. 1710D. Traumatic Brain Injury: Comprehensive Program for Long-Term Rehabilitation.

f. Title 38 U.S.C. 1710E. Traumatic Brain Injury: Use of Non-Department Facilities for Rehabilitation.

g. VHA Handbook 1170.01.

h. VHA Handbook 1010.01.

i. VHA Handbook 1601B.05.

j. *Memorandum of Agreement* (MOA) between VA and DOD on Referral of Active Duty Military Personnel Who Sustain Spinal Cord Injury, Traumatic Brain Injury, or Blindness to Veterans Affairs Facilities for Health Care and Rehabilitative Services, December 13, 2006.

k. Veterans Health Initiative, Traumatic Brain Injury; January 2004.

6. FOLLOW-UP RESPONSIBILITIES:
The Chief Consultant, Rehabilitation Services, within the office of Patient Care Services, has overall responsibility for the contents of this Directive. Questions may be referred to the PM&RS National Director at (612) 725-2044. Facsimile transmission may be sent to (612) 727-5642.

7. RESCISSIONS:
VHA Directive 2005-024, dated June 8, 2005, is rescinded. This VHA Directive expires June 30, 2014.

Gerald M. Cross, MD, FAAFP
Acting Under Secretary for Health

DISTRIBUTION: CO: E-mailed 6/11/09
                  FLD: VISN, MA, DO, OC,CRO, and 200 – E-mailed

6/11/09FLD:

Attachment A. Required* Core Dedicated Staffing Per Twelve Beds for Each Polytrauma-Traumatic Brain Injury (TBI) Rehabilitation Center

DISCIPLINE	Full-time Equivalent (FTE)
Rehabilitation Physician	1
Nurse Manager	1
Registered Nurse (2.0 must be Certified Rehabilitation Registered Nurse (CRRN)	11
Licensed Practical Nurse and/or Certified Nursing Assistant	8
Nurse Educator	1
Clinical Nurse Leader (CNL)**	1
Admission and Follow-up Nurse Case Manager	1
Social Worker	3
Speech-Language Pathologist	3
Physical Therapist	3.5
Occupational Therapist	3.5
Recreation Therapist	2
Neuropsychologist	1
Counseling Psychologist	1
Family Therapist	1
Blind Rehabilitation Outpatient Specialist	1
Certified Prosthetist	1
Certified Driver Trainer	1
Program Administrator	1
Program Assistant	1

* Variances from the staffing model must be approved by the Physical Medicine and Rehabilitation Service Program Office.

** The CNL is a mandated position for all patient care settings in all VA medical centers by 2016 and the rapid implementation of this role in the polytrauma-TBI network is a high priority. The Office of Nursing Service will assist sites, as needed, with the implementation.

Attachment B. Polytrauma-Traumatic Brain Injury (TBI) Transitional Rehabilitation Program (PTRP) Required Core Staffing

DISCIPLINES	Full-time Equivalent (FTE)
Program Director	1
Program Assistant	1
Physiatrist	.5
Psychiatrist	.5
Registered Nurse	1
Licensed Practical Nurse	5
Speech Language Pathologist	1
Occupational Therapist	2
Physical Therapist	.5
Recreation Therapist	2
Recreation Therapist Assistant	1
Neuropsychologist	1
Counseling Psychologist	1
Social Worker	1
Blind Rehabilitation Outpatient Specialist	.5

Attachment C. Dedicated Consultative Services Recommended at Each Medical Center with a Polytrauma-Traumatic Brain Injury (TBI) Rehabilitation Center

Audiology
Cardiology
Clinical Nutrition
Clinical Chaplain
Clinical Pharmacy
Dentistry and/or Oral and Maxillofacial Surgery
Driver Training
Ear, Nose, and Throat (ENT)
Endocrinology

Attachment C (Continued)

Gastroenterology
General Internal Medicine
General Surgery
Infectious Disease
Neurology
Neuroophthalmology
Neurosurgery
Optometry
Orthopedic Surgery
Plastic Surgery
Psychiatry
Post-traumatic Stress Disorder (PTSD) Clinic Team
Pulmonary
Radiology
Urology
Vocational Rehabilitation

Attachment D. Polytrauma Network Site Required Core Staffing

DISCIPLINES	Full-time Equivalent (FTE)
Rehabilitation Physician	.5*
Rehabilitation Nurse	.5*
Social Worker	.5*
Speech-Language Pathologist	.5*
Physical Therapist	.5*
Occupational Therapist	.5*
Psychologist	.5*
Blind Rehabilitation Outpatient Specialist	.5
Certified Prosthetist	.5

* A minimum of .5 FTE is required, however, increases need to be made based on workload demands.

Polytrauma Network Site Additional Staff Recommended

DISCIPLINE	Full-time Equivalent (FTE)
Program Manager	*
Program Assistant	*
Patient Family Clinical Educator	*
Therapeutic Recreation Specialist	*
Vocational Specialist	*
Other Disciplines based on local needs	*

* FTE is determined by workload demand.

Attachment E. Polytrauma Support Clinic Team Required Core Staffing

DISCIPLINE	Full-time Equivalent (FTE)
Rehabilitation Physician	.5*
Rehabilitation Nurse	.5*
Social Worker	.5*
Speech-Language Pathologist	.5*
Physical Therapist	.5*
Occupational Therapist	.5*
Psychologist	.5*
Other Disciplines based on local needs	

* A minimum of .5 FTE is required, however, increases need to be made based on workload demands.

Attachment F

Regional Polytrauma-Traumatic Brain Injury (TBI) Rehabilitation Center	Veterans Integrated Service Network (VISN)	Polytrauma TBI Network Site	Polytrauma-TBI Support Clinic Teams	Polytrauma-TBI Point of Contact

			(Continued)	
Richmond	VISN 1	Boston	West Haven Togus White River Northampton	Bedford Manchester Providence
	VISN 2	Syracuse	Albany Buffalo Bath Canandaigua	
	VISN 3	Bronx	Hudson Valley Health Care System (HCS) at Montrose Hudson Valley HCS at Castle Point NJ (New Jersey) HCS at East Orange NJHCS at Lyons NY (New York) Harbor HCS at New York NY Harbor HCS at Brooklyn NY Harbor HCS at St Albans Northport VA Medical Center	
	VISN 4	Philadelphia	Pittsburgh Wilmington Erie Lebanon Coatesville Altoona Butler Wilkes-Barre	Clarksburg
	VISN 5	Washington DC	Baltimore Martinsburg	
	VISN 6	Richmond	Hampton Salisbury Durham	Asheville Beckley Fayetteville Salem
Tampa	VISN 7	Augusta	Tuscaloosa Columbia Charleston Atlanta Birmingham	Dublin Tuskegee

	VISN 8	Tampa San Juan	Bay Pines Gainesville Miami West Palm	Orlando
	VISN 9	Lexington	Huntington Louisville Memphis Tennessee Valley (TV) Health Care (HC) at Nashville TVHC at Murfreesboro Mountain Home	
	VISN 16	Houston	Alexandria Jackson Central Arkansas-Little Rock Gulf Coast (Biloxi) Fayetteville, AR Oklahoma City Muskogee Shreveport	New Orleans
	VISN 17	Dallas	Temple San Antonio	Waco Kerrville
Palo Alto	VISN 18	Southern Arizona HCS (Tucson)	New Mexico HCS at Albuquerque	Amarillo West Texas HCS (Big Spring) El Paso Northern Arizona HCS (Prescott) Phoenix
	VISN 19	Denver	Salt Lake Grand Junction	Cheyenne Montana HCS at Ft. Harrison Sheridan

(Continued)

	VISN 20	Seattle	Portland Boise	Alaska American Lake Roseburg Spokane Walla Walla White City
	VISN 21	Palo Alto	Sacramento San Francisco	Sierra Nevada HCS Honolulu Manila Central California HCS (Fresno)
	VISN 22	West LA	Long Beach San Diego Loma Linda	Southern Nevada HCS Sepulveda
Minneapolis	VISN 10	Cleveland	Cincinnati Dayton	Columbus Chillicothe
	VISN 11	Indianapolis	Detroit Danville (Indiana) Ann Arbor	Battle Creek Northern Indiana Health Care System (NIHCS) at Marion Saginaw
	VISN 12	Hines	Milwaukee North Chicago Tomah Madison Chicago HCS (Jesse Brown)	Iron Mountain
	VISN 15	St. Louis	Kansas City	Wichita Poplar Bluff Columbia MO Eastern Kansas at Topeka Marion

| | VISN 23 | Minneapolis | Sioux Falls
Black Hills
Iowa City
Central Iowa at Knoxville
St Cloud | Fargo
Central Iowa at Des Moines
Greater Nebraska at Grand Island
Greater Nebraska at Lincoln
Omaha |

Chapter Sources

The following chapters have been previously published:

Chapter 1 – This is an edited, excerpted and augmented edition of a United States Congressional Research Service publication, Report Order Code R40941, dated November 25, 2009.

Chapter 2 – This is an edited, excerpted and augmented edition of a National Council on Disability publication, dated March 4, 2009.

Chapter 3 – This is an edited, excerpted and augmented edition of a United States Government Accountability Office publication, Report Order Code GAO-09-108, dated January 2009.

Chapter 4 –This is an edited, excerpted and augmented edition of a Department of Veteran Affairs publication, Report Order Code 2009-028, dated J

Index

N

O

P